About the Author

A former project manager in the nuclear industry, James Titcombe became involved in patient safety following the tragic loss of his baby son due to failures in his care at Morecambe Bay Trust in 2008.

Working with other families, he successfully campaigned for the Morecambe Bay Investigation which was published in March 2015.

In 2013 he began work as the National Advisor on Safety for the Care Quality Commission.

He regularly speaks at national conferences on the subject of patient safety and has had articles published in healthcare journals as well as the national press.

James is a Patron of the charity Action against Medical Accidents (AvMA).

In 2015 James was awarded an OBE for services to patient safety.

Joshua's Story

James Titcombe

Uncovering the
Morecambe Bay
NHS scandal

Joshua's Story - Uncovering the Morecambe Bay NHS scandal

© James Titcombe 2015

Cover and book design by Jane Dixon-Smith
Edited by Roland Denning and Murray Anderson-Wallace

Print ISBN 978-0-9934492-0-8
Ebook-Mobi ISBN 978-0-9934492-1-5
Ebook-ePub ISBN 978-0-9934492-2-2

Anderson Wallace Publishing
5 Ancaster Road
Leeds LS16 5HH

Printed and bound in the UK by Clays, St Ives PLC

In memory of our much loved and badly missed baby boy, Joshua, and all those who tragically lost their lives in the Morecambe Bay NHS scandal.

Contents

Foreword

There is no greater love than that of a father for his son and that is what this book is ultimately about. It's the struggle by one man to deliver justice for his son and his family but, in the process, James Titcombe reveals a tragedy that affected many other families and unravelled one of the most significant scandals in UK healthcare, reaching to the top of the NHS.

In many ways the National Health Service is still coming to terms with the reality of what happened to parents and babies on the maternity ward at Furness General Hospital over a period of almost nine years. This includes having to accept how some of the most powerful organisations and figures at the top of the health system avoided taking the necessary and vital action to step in and ensure patient safety despite clear and numerous opportunities to do so. There have been and will continue to be substantial changes to the NHS, specifically in maternity care but also in the wider agenda of patient safety, as a result of what we now know about events at the University Hospitals of Morecambe Bay Foundation Trust. The genesis of some of these changes began with James Titcombe's campaign on behalf of his son. While the work goes on, for many of the families who fought for so long to get to the truth, the healing has only just started.

In 2008 when his son Joshua died James Titcombe, like so many bereaved fathers, simply had questions that needed answers. His family were grieving and what should have been the happiest of times was enveloped in darkness. How many of us would have the strength and resolve at a time like that to pursue the truth? The story of Joshua and his father's journey over the following seven years, exposing first the poor care at the hospital and the failure of its management, before going on to expose the negligence of the wider NHS regulatory system, is essential reading for anyone looking to understand how a service like the NHS, so revered as it is by the public, can let down those who most rely on it. This story is a glimpse into the extraordinary lengths families are sometimes forced to go to in order to obtain justice for their loved ones and why the public at large owe them a debt of gratitude that will largely never be repaid.

I first spoke to James Titcombe in 2012 and was immediately struck by his personal honesty and integrity. James has a sharp mind and a forensic ability to sort fact from fiction, a skill he has used to great effect over the years. James and I worked together on a number of articles exploring and picking holes in the official record of how problems at Morecambe Bay were not properly investigated by regulators, despite them having clear knowledge of what had gone wrong. It was James' ability to sift through hundreds of documents and explore every avenue that produced some of the most fertile grounds for further investigation of the issues. His determination to force the release of internal documents revealed the true failure of some of the national NHS organisations; exposing a culture not of patient safety and high quality care but of meeting targets, ticking the box regardless of the outcomes for patients.

At almost every turn there was denial, obfuscation and dishonesty but James met all of this with a steely resolve armed with facts and evidence that eventually overwhelmed the deniers and led to the creation of the Morecambe Bay Investigation chaired by Dr Bill Kirkup. That inquiry's findings, published in March 2015, laid bare the truth about what was really happening on the wards at Furness General Hospital years before the death of baby Joshua. It described in detail the attitude and culture that prevailed among the group of so-called 'musketeer midwives' whose catalogue of incidents and failings are even now difficult to understand or reconcile with that of a caring profession. Worse still, the investigation detailed the missed opportunities and failures in national regulators and government policy that contributed to what happened. It detailed a 'lethal mix' of failings at every level of the NHS which ultimately contributed to the avoidable deaths of 11 babies and one mother – ripping apart those families' lives forever.

There is a tremendous amount of learning in the pages of this book and for me as a journalist, working with families who have suffered poor care, what strikes me about the story of Joshua and the families of Morecambe Bay is again the level to which they had to go to get the answers they needed. Reflecting on their journey over the last decade, it's hard to appreciate the anguish that going up against the bureaucracy of the NHS causes people. It starts almost immediately with the local hospital investigation and continues right the way through to the Parliamentary Health Service Ombudsman.

Sadly this was not isolated to Morecambe Bay and is evident in far too many cases of patient harm in the health service. This lack of an open and transparent culture was a shadow hanging over Stafford Hospital where I worked with families to expose appalling standards of care and routine neglect of hundreds of patients from 2008 onwards, just a few years before the events at Morecambe Bay became more widely known. Staffordshire families were told their experiences were a one-off, the result of local management failings, and that claims of a systematic cultural problem in the NHS were farfetched. But then came James Titcombe and the families from Morecambe Bay. This book underlines the fatal complacency and unwillingness to accept that the NHS could make mistakes that existed at the time. What these scandals show is that there was and, indeed, may still be a cultural and systemic failure within the NHS to look into the mirror and see its true self and take action. We shouldn't have to rely on heroic efforts by grieving parents and loved-ones to show us the truth they have had to learn so painfully on our behalf.

The NHS is an amazing national icon. What it stands for - free universal healthcare to all regardless of ability to pay - is, I believe, one of the single greatest accomplishments Britain achieved in the last century. Day in and day out doctors, nurses and hundreds of other types of staff work incredibly hard to deliver the ideals the NHS was founded on. It sees around one million patients every 36 hours and the vast majority receive great care delivered by staff with compassion and competence in a system that is one of the most efficient in the world.

But let's not pretend the NHS doesn't make mistakes. In fact it makes a lot: 1.47 million patient safety incidents were recorded across the NHS between April 2013 and March 2014 with a total of 3,785 resulting in a death – 10 deaths a day. Healthcare is a human endeavour, delivered by people who, quite understandably, sometimes make mistakes. But it is how the NHS responds to those mistakes which reveals whether we have the right culture in our wards and hospitals. What the story of Joshua and Morecambe Bay shows us is that the NHS sometimes compounds its mistakes by trying to hide the fact they happened in the first place. Morecambe

Bay wasn't the first NHS scandal, it won't be the last. Families who find themselves up against this culture are often broken by it; first betrayed by a service they are taught to cherish and trust and then chewed up by the same service which refuses to acknowledge any wrongdoing. The NHS must stop destroying the lives of bereaved families who deserve the truth about what happened to their loved ones. It's a challenge the NHS must rise to meet.

In the last few years, in no small part thanks to patient advocates like James Titcombe, progress has been made. There has been a clear recognition of the need to be more open and transparent about errors and mistakes and, while we are far from saying mission accomplished, safety is now more than ever on the agenda. Development of new duty of candour laws around honesty with families when incidents occur and a better focus on patient safety at board level are important steps on the path to a better NHS but, as always, the financial and political pressures that pull and twist the NHS from the sidelines forever threaten what achievements there have been.

New laws and tougher regulatory sanctions by themselves won't deliver an improved culture in the NHS. The responsibility rests with each and every member of the 1.4m staff who work in the NHS from the cleaners to the chief executives.

A helpful start to changing the NHS culture is to be honest with ourselves about where we have come from and where we need to go. I hope Joshua's story is read far and wide by those both in the NHS and outside of it. I hope it helps people to understand and change their own behaviour. I hope it will be a catalyst to help us reach a better place.

Shaun Lintern

Shaun Lintern is an investigative journalist who has worked with families to expose poor care at both Stafford Hospital and Morecambe Bay. He is patient safety correspondent at the Health Service Journal.

Introduction

It's 2002 and I'm on the back of a motorbike in the heat and dirt of Vietnam, being driven round the exotic sights of Hanoi. But this is no holiday; I'm here for six months, working for an engineering construction company building and commissioning new coal-fired power stations. The year before I'd graduated in engineering, so this is a great and exciting opportunity for me in many ways.

The driver of the motorbike is Hoa, an enchanting woman I've just met who already seems to be playing a very import-ant role in my life. Hoa is an economics graduate from Hanoi and it is soon clear that this is more than just sightseeing. We meet most weekends and we begin to fall in love.

Two years later we are married and in 2005 our daughter Emily is born. We buy our first house, a small two-bedroom terrace in the town of Dalton-in-Furness, not far from where my parents live in Cumbria.

We're happily married and life seems perfect. On October 27th, 2008, our second child, Joshua, is born at Furness General Hospital - a perfect baby boy.

But soon our world is torn apart. After eight days of fighting for his life in intensive care, Joshua dies at the Freeman Hospital in Newcastle.

This book is the story of a six year battle to uncover the truth about what happened to Joshua and why he came to die from a condition that could have easily been prevented with the most basic of medical care.

Joshua's death was not an isolated event; during this long journey I discovered that many other lives had been lost through similar failures in care. Something had to be done but everywhere I turned to for help led to a closed door. With the help of some exceptional people at key moments, the full truth about Joshua's death and the catastrophic failures in maternity care at Furness General Hospital eventually emerged. The difficulties I confronted in trying to learn the truth about Joshua's death were faced by many other people unfortunate enough to find themselves in similar positions.

The problems at the Morecambe Bay NHS Foundation Trust have been subject to much media coverage, but I wanted to write this book to tell a personal story from beginning to end, from the inside, as it happened to me and my family.

I hope this book will be read by patients, parents, healthcare professionals and politicians. There needs to be a transformation in the way healthcare organisations respond to incidents of avoidable harm and learn from error. I hope this book can be part of that process.

An encouraging drive in the NHS has begun to improve transparency and safety – it is vital that this continues.

Chapter 1 - The short life and death of Joshua Titcombe

It is early 2008 and I've just had some wonderful news - my wife Hoa is pregnant with our second child. I can't wait to share the news with my parents and Emily, our three-year-old daughter. When we discover the baby is going to be a boy we talk about calling him John. A few days later I'm having my hair cut in town and talking to the hairdresser about baby names. The name Joshua comes up. The hairdresser likes the name and so do I; in my mind this is what I want to call my new son. Hoa agrees and, much to Emily's disappointment, John becomes Joshua.

The pregnancy goes well. Hoa is the perfect mother-to-be, determinedly keeping fit and eating healthy organic food. Hoa's mum is coming over from Vietnam to visit us. We've recently moved house and we do everything we can to make the baby's room as nice as possible including, as expectant parents do, a collection of cute baby clothes ready for Joshua's arrival. The new member of our family will be here in time for Christmas.

In the week of October 20th, 2008 our excitement has been slightly tempered - the whole family has been feeling poorly

1

for several days. Emily has been sent home from nursery and Hoa and I have sore throats and headaches. I finish work on Friday 24th, relieved to have the weekend to recuperate.

On Saturday night at about 9pm I hear Hoa shouting from the bathroom. Her waters have broken. Trying to stay calm, I phone my mum and tell her what is happening. She tells us to call the Maternity Unit and arrange to go in. My mum warns us about the risk of infection and how we must be sure to tell the staff that we have been feeling poorly.

During Emily's birth I had felt anxious and worried. The experience had been stressful but the outcome, despite my concern, was wonderful. I know a bit more about childbirth now and I promise myself that, this time, I'm going to be more relaxed and place my trust in the staff. My role will be to stay calm and reassure Hoa. I want her to be as relaxed and confident as possible. These thoughts are going through my head as I drive Hoa to the Maternity Unit at Furness General Hospital on Saturday 25th.

When we arrive the Unit is expecting us. Hoa is upset and crying. The midwives ask her what's wrong and she explains that she's been feeling poorly for several days, she's had a headache and a sore throat. I tell them I've been feeling ill too. Hoa is tired and anxious. We're told there's nothing to be worried about and that the illness is probably a virus - 'there's a lot going around'.

My wife is exactly 37 weeks pregnant. NICE guidelines recommend that any woman whose waters break before 37 weeks should be given precautionary antibiotics prior to labour to mitigate against the increased risk of infection, but we don't know this at the time. We're not given antibiotics. Instead, we are reassured that everything is fine. The midwives

2

take temperatures and monitor for contractions - there are none. The foetal heart rate is monitored. We're given advice about monitoring Hoa's temperature and checking on the colour of fluids and then sent home. We're told to come back if the contractions start or, if not, the next morning for another check up as 'we don't do inductions at the weekend'.

Throughout the night nothing happens, so we go back to the Maternity Unit the next day. The same checks are carried out and again we're advised to go home and wait for contractions to start and, if they don't, to come back the following day. We go home then drive to my mum and dad's house and go for a walk in an attempt to spur the contractions on. Nothing happens. We go for an evening meal in a local pub, but still no contractions. We go home and have an early night, by this time getting a little anxious. In the early hours of Monday morning, at around 5am, the contractions begin.

My parents come round straight away. I phone the hospital who tell us to wait until the contractions are closer together. This happens very soon and at 6.30am I drive Hoa to the hospital. She is quickly assessed and almost immediately transferred to a labour room - and just in time.

Joshua is born at 7.38am on Monday, October 27th, 2008.

As Joshua is being delivered, the midwife suggests that I cut the cord but, when Joshua is born, he is very blue, floppy and appears not to be breathing. The midwife takes over and cuts the cord and Joshua is taken straight away to a small table at the side of Hoa's bed and placed on his back. I'm worried, but the midwife tells me everything is OK and starts to rub his chest saying, 'Come on little fellow'. Still nothing. Joshua is blue, limp and unresponsive. There's more rubbing of his chest. By now Hoa is uneasy and asking what's wrong. The midwife tells me she's going to take Joshua out of the room to give him some oxygen to 'get him started'. She says I can go with her so, anxiously, I follow Joshua and the midwife into a small side room. The door to the birth room is left open. Joshua is given a short blast of oxygen with a facial mask. He immediately lets out a big cry and starts to breathe. I tell the midwife I must go and tell Hoa. She tells me I don't need to worry - Hoa would have heard the cry. She had. We are both relieved. Joshua is carried back into the room. His colour is much better. He is pink and looks healthy. Hoa has her first cuddle and we both have tears of pride in our eyes.

I know all parents must feel this way about their babies, but Joshua really is a perfect and beautiful little boy. All my worries are over - Joshua has been born and we have all the time in the world to get to know our baby son.

Joshua is wrapped up in a blanket and put in his cot. He was born just as the night shift was finishing so the midwives who delivered him disappear soon after his birth. We are left alone. I take some photos of Joshua in his cot and phone my parents to tell them the good news. Then I hold Joshua in my arms and give him a long cuddle.

About 30 minutes later Hoa tells me that she feels very cold and unwell. I put my coat over her but she quickly gets worse. She starts to shake and asks me to get help. I'm very worried. With Joshua in my arms I go out in to the Maternity Unit to look for help.

The ward is quiet and it takes a few minutes before I find someone. When I do, the midwife is concerned that I carried Joshua out of the room. She says I was wrong to do that – it's a health and safety issue. I explain what is happening to Hoa and the midwife comes with me back to the room. Joshua is returned to his cot.

By this stage Hoa is clearly very unwell. Her eyes roll to the back of her head and she is barely responsive. The midwife tries to take her blood pressure but the machine doesn't appear to be working. She takes her temperature – it's very high. The midwife says she will call for some fluids and antibiotics and leaves.

After what seems like a very long time, but is probably only around 15 minutes, the midwife arrives with an overhead drip, telling me she is going to cannulise Hoa and start the fluids. She says the antibiotics are on their way. The midwife has trouble inserting the cannula (a hollow needle inserted into a vein to administer medication), but eventually manages it and the drip starts. The antibiotics arrive about 10 minutes later. When they do, the midwife can't insert the second cannula at all. Help is summoned and, a short while later, a junior doctor arrives on the scene. He can't insert the cannula either so a second doctor is called. He manages to get the cannula in and the antibiotic drip is set to work. As the doctor leaves, I stop him and ask if Joshua might also need antibiotics - would he look and make sure he was OK? The doctor gives me a nervous look, waves his hand dismissively and leaves the room.

I ask the midwives whether or not there was any risk that Joshua might also need antibiotics. The response I get back is clear and absolute.

> 'Joshua is absolutely fine. It's your wife you need to be concerned about.'

> 'My wife needs antibiotics, why doesn't Joshua?'

> 'The infection in Hoa is in a different system. We know Joshua is fine just by looking at him.'

Why don't I take issue with these explanations? Why am I not screaming at the top of my lungs at this point? Shouldn't I be running out of the labour room and demanding to see the person in charge? Should I be insisting a paediatrician comes to see Joshua and assess him? How can I make sense of all of this?

I think about the birth of Emily – it seemed horrific to me, yet the outcome was a healthy and beautiful baby girl. Who am I to be anxious about Joshua when he is being cared for by professional staff who see newborn babies every day and know what they are doing? I want to trust, I *need* to trust the experts who are looking after my newborn son.

Two hours later, Hoa seems to have made a good recovery. It's a huge relief when she opens her eyes and talks. She asks about Joshua. She's deeply concerned, but I pass on the reassurance I've been given by the midwives - Joshua is fine. Hoa is still anxious and wants me to ask about Joshua again. Around midday a midwife comes in to the room and tells us that we are going to be moved to the postnatal ward. I ask again about Joshua. I explain how Hoa and I had been feeling ill before the birth, that Hoa's waters had been broken for two days before Joshua was born and that Hoa collapsed after the birth with a fever and needed antibiotics and fluids.

The midwife tells me that she will phone the paediatricians and make sure a doctor comes to look at Joshua. The midwife goes off and, a short while later, another midwife comes to move us into the postnatal ward. Hoa is put into a wheelchair and Joshua is pushed in his cot. As we are walking along the corridor we're told we are going to be placed in a small room with 'isolation' written on the door, but we shouldn't worry, because the only reason for this is that the main postnatal ward is full. Then the midwife who previously told me she was going to ask the paediatricians to review Joshua appears on the scene.

> 'I've phoned the paediatricians but they're very busy,' she tells me. 'Don't worry, we're going to monitor Joshua very closely every hour to make sure he is OK.'

Why do I accept this? Why don't I insist something more is done? The answer again is trust. I trust what I am told and I know that if there was any chance Joshua is at any kind of risk, the staff will take action.

Once in the small room labelled 'isolation', Hoa and I are left alone. No one calls in to check on us. Hoa starts to get anxious - Joshua hasn't been fed. Hoa asks me if it is safe to breastfeed Joshua, given that she collapsed with an infection. I tell her I'll try to find a midwife to ask.

When I leave the room I can't see anyone immediately around, but there's an open door ahead of me down the corridor. As I walk towards it I see a group of midwives inside the room chatting and drinking tea. I put my head round the door and ask if I could speak to someone. They're not pleased to see me. I ask a midwife if she was aware of my wife and Joshua and their recent history. She doesn't seem to know. I explain how my wife and I were unwell before the labour, that her waters had broken two days before Joshua was born, that she'd collapsed after the birth and needed antibiotics and fluids. The midwife says she knew all this. I ask why no one has been to see Joshua - I had understood Joshua was going to be monitored every hour. She tells me, crossly, I'm wrong - Joshua will be monitored every three hours and that someone will be along shortly.

A while later a maternity assistant comes into our room. We ask if it is OK to breastfeed Joshua. She says she'll feed him with formula and a syringe. I help her feed Joshua. He's mucousy, sleepy and lethargic and not at all interested in taking the milk. We ask about Joshua's condition and we are told that it's normal for newborn babies to be like this.

Over the next 18 hours, Joshua continues to be lethargic and mucousy, but another concern arises. His temperature is measured several times and found to be very low. The recorded temperatures are written on a bright yellow observation chart, kept by Joshua's cot. Hoa clearly remembers reading two of the temperatures on this chart. One is 36.1° and the other 35.8°.

In response to his low temperatures, Joshua is moved into a heated cot. At one point an overhead radiant heater is placed directly above him. Hoa asks me if he is OK and not too hot. The midwife in the room overhears. She puts her hand on Joshua's skin and, feeling how hot he is, quickly pulls the overhead heater away saying, 'We don't want to cook him, do we?'

Throughout the rest of the day and night we are told that Joshua's temperature is too low. On at least three occasions he is transferred to a different cot with some form of heating. The fact that Joshua has a low temperature and not a high temperature reassures me that he doesn't have his mother's infection. I discuss this with the midwife:

> 'At least we can relax about infection, can't we, as Joshua's temperature is low and not high?'

> She pats me on the back and says, 'That's right Mr Titcombe, Joshua is just fine.'

In the afternoon my parents come to visit, bringing Emily with them. My mum gives Joshua a cuddle with a look of

8

pride and happiness on her face. We take a photo of Emily holding Joshua, other nervous hands around him making sure he is safe. I go home for the night and make plans to bring Joshua home the next day.

The next morning I'm at home, the baby seat is in the car and the cot ready in Joshua's room. At around 9am I get a phone call from the Maternity Ward. I'm not told much, only that Joshua is having trouble with his breathing and that my wife is very upset. I phone my mum and tell her what I've been told. I hear a gasp down the phone and she starts to cry. I tell her not to worry, it's probably nothing serious, but I need mum and dad to come around to look after Emily so I can go straight to the hospital. Within 10 minutes my parents arrive. I don't say much, but rush to the car and drive off.

By the time I arrive at Furness General Hospital, Joshua is in the Special Care Baby Unit. Hoa is sitting in a side room in floods of tears. She's had a terrible night – still in pain from the birth and very worried about the grunting sounds that Joshua has been making. I try to comfort her and reassure her that everything will be OK, then I go to see Joshua. He is with a doctor and other nurses, breathing with his own lungs but with assisted oxygen through small tubes in his nostrils. A few moments later, the doctor tells me he needs to be fully ventilated and I'm asked to leave the room. Around this time my dad arrives. He and I hug and we both cry. A young midwife looks at us both, shakes her head then tuts:

> 'Haven't you been through anything like this before?'

> 'No,' I reply, 'I haven't.'

Throughout the next few hours we know Joshua's condition is serious, but we're not given a clear picture of what's wrong.

9

The doctor suspects Joshua has a heart problem. Then later he tells us that Joshua has something wrong with his oesophagus and needs some sort of corrective surgery. A transfer team will be coming down from Manchester.

The team from Manchester arrive and set to work to stabilise Joshua for transfer. The reality of the situation hasn't sunk in yet; we are all confused and in shock. The first time the scale of what is happening hits home is when a transfer nurse takes me to a side room to talk. She tells me that Joshua is in a very serious condition and, if he survives, we have to be aware of the possibility that his oxygen levels may have dipped enough to cause serious brain damage.

Within the space of a few hours I've gone from the anticipation and joy of preparing to take home a healthy baby son to being faced with the possibility that Joshua could die or survive with serious disability. I don't want to believe what I'm being told. My world has turned upside down. I am devastated.

I have a conversation with another transfer nurse called Andy. He talks to me about what they think is wrong with Joshua. When they swapped his ventilation tubes there were brown sticky secretions that looked like meconium - this is the substance that babies produce with their first bowel movements. Andy explains that this could be one of Joshua's problems. I tell him about the history of the birth and mention that Joshua had been very cold during the day and night and needed to be repeatedly heated.

> Andy looks at me and says, 'A low temperature
> is a classic sign of infection in newborn babies.'

I'm stunned. Joshua repeatedly had a low temperature. If this is a classic sign of infection in babies, why hadn't someone referred Joshua to a doctor and given him antibiotics earlier?

From that moment I am acutely aware that something has gone very badly wrong at Furness General Hospital. I can't quite believe what is happening - it seems neither real nor possible. I want to scream as loudly as I can and demand answers there and then, but our focus has to be on Joshua. More than anything else, we want him to pull through so we can take him home.

In the late evening the transfer team is ready to take Joshua by ambulance to Manchester. We're told we can't travel with him and that we'll have to make our own way. Hoa is discharged, still with the cannulas from the drips sticking in her arms, still bleeding from the birth and in pain. We make arrangements for my parents to look after Emily and, at around 10.30pm, we set off by car for Manchester St Mary's Hospital.

I'm not in a fit state to drive, barely able to focus on the motorway ahead. I'm doing 45 miles per hour in the inside lane with cars beeping behind. We pull into Lancaster Services and I tell Hoa I can't drive any further - we need to get a room in the Travelodge and rest for the night. Hoa is hysterical and screams that she doesn't want to leave Joshua alone. She wants to be with her son. I go to the service area shop and buy two cans of Red Bull and some caffeine strips - the kind you put on your tongue to dissolve. We carry on with the journey and eventually arrive at St Mary's Hospital in the early hours of the morning of Wednesday 29th October.

We go straight to the Paediatric Intensive Care Unit where we're greeted by a kind and softly spoken nurse who tells us about Joshua's current state. The blood samples taken from Joshua in Barrow showed that he had overwhelming

11

pneumococcus infection, the same infection that Hoa had collapsed from shortly after Joshua's birth. There is nothing wrong with Joshua's oesophagus and his heart is healthy. This confirms all our concerns about FGH. How could this have happened? But now isn't the time for questions. We have to concentrate on Joshua.

A consultant is called in the middle of the night to manage Joshua's intensive care. Joshua is on a ventilator receiving maximum life support. His oxygen levels are being monitored and his saturation, the measure of how much oxygen is in his blood, is acceptable and steady. However, if Joshua's condition deteriorates, there is no Plan B.

The ventilator is turned up as high as possible and is putting pressure on Joshua's heart. For the first time we first hear the term 'ECMO'. ECMO stands for Extra Corporeal Membrane Oxygenation. In simple terms, this is a heart and lung machine. ECMO treatment would involve Joshua's blood being taken outside his body and pumped around a machine that does the job the lungs normally do to oxygenate the blood. This would allow Joshua's lungs to rest and recover from the infection, at which point the ECMO machine would slowly be wound down to allow Joshua's own lungs to take over.

But there are risks. ECMO involves taking the blood outside the body through a series of tubes. To avoid blood clots a drug called Heptin is needed to thin the blood. This increases the risk of internal bleeding, including to the brain. The risks are explained to us in figures: 80% of babies survive ECMO and make a recovery, although often with other problems, including brain damage.

At about 3am we leave Joshua and try to get some rest. We're taken to a small room with a single bed. Hoa still has cannulas sticking out from her arms. I ask the nurse if I could have a paracetamol. She tells me it's against the rules as I'm not a patient. I lie down on the cold floor at the side of Hoa's bed. Neither of us sleep.

At around 7am we go to see Joshua again. His oxygen levels have been stable during the night, but he still needs maximum life support. The stress this would be putting on his heart is emphasised and the option of ECMO raised again. There are a number of specialist centres in the UK that could provide ECMO and the Manchester team were contacting them. Hoa and I are scared and unsure. I phone my parents and explain the situation. They're unsure too. My brother-in-law, Nik, a university lecturer from Leeds, arranges to come to Manchester to meet us at the hospital. He arrives mid-morning. By this time Hoa has seen a midwife; the cannulas in her arm have been removed and her stitches checked.

We ask to speak to the consultant about ECMO. Nik, Hoa and I go into a small side room to have the conversation. We talk in depth about Joshua's condition and what the options are. In the end, I ask the consultant the only question we really need answered.

'If Joshua was your son, what would you do?'

The response comes without hesitation. 'I would put my son on ECMO'.

From that moment we don't feel we have a choice. If we refuse the opportunity to put Joshua on ECMO and he dies we would never forgive ourselves. We agree that this is the right thing to do.

We're told a team from the Freeman Hospital in Newcastle will be transferring Joshua by helicopter. The transfer team arrives mid-afternoon and we're taken through the consent forms. We sign the forms confirming that, as Joshua's parents, we understand the risks and authorise Joshua to be placed on ECMO at Newcastle. I make one request. I understand ECMO to be the Plan B and, if Joshua's condition deteriorates further, there won't be another backup plan. I ask the transfer team to make sure Joshua is not put on ECMO in Newcastle unless he really needs to be. I ask for an assurance that my wife and I will be phoned before such a decision is made. This is agreed.

Joshua is stabilised by the Newcastle team and transferred by helicopter to the Freeman Hospital. Nik, Hoa and I follow in our car. An hour into the journey my mobile phone rings and I pull in to the side of the road. It's the Newcastle team. Joshua has arrived safely but the Newcastle consultant feels that he needs to be put on ECMO straight away. His oxygen levels are stable but he is receiving maximum life support and his body is under stress. We're told that ECMO is Joshua's best chance of survival; the consultant feels that this is closer to 90% than 80% in his case. I ask Hoa and Nik what they think. We all agree that we have to follow the advice we've been given. We continue with the journey and arrive at the Freeman Hospital about two hours later.

When we arrive a member of the transfer team is just leaving the hospital. She recognises us and immediately reassures us that Joshua is fine. He has been transferred to ECMO successfully and is doing well. She gives us directions to the Paediatric Intensive Care Unit. There we are greeted by the consultant looking after Joshua on the Unit. She is the kind of person who instils an instant sense of trust; she speaks factually, but empathetically and kindly. She is clearly passionate about her work. She discusses Joshua's condition at length and shows us photos and letters from the families of babies and children who have been treated by ECMO in the past and made a recovery.

We then go to see Joshua. We're warned that there would be a lot of equipment, but we're still shocked when we see him. He is cocooned in wires and tubes with electrode patches, each printed with a teddy bear's face, placed all over his body. Despite this, Joshua looks comfortable and at rest. He is under a lot of sedation so his eyes are closed, but his little hand is moving up towards his mouth. If you put your finger in his hand, he grips it like babies do.

This is how we see Joshua over the next seven days: cold, sedated and hooked up to machines supporting his life. We want desperately to pick him up and cuddle him. As parents we are scared, anxious and desperately wanting to take our little boy home.

We are given accommodation in a flat within the grounds of the hospital. Over the next few days we start to get into a routine. There's a small room in the children's ward where mothers can express milk for their babies. When we are not by Joshua's side or sleeping, we spend time there. We nickname the room the 'therapy room', because that's what it is for us. Hoa is able to express milk for Joshua and we have conversations with some of the lovely and supportive children's nurses on the ward. Talking helps.

The next five days are positive. Although desperately worried and anxious, our main concern is for Joshua's brain condition. The thought that we could lose him has been pushed far back in our minds. On November 3rd, 2008, things change. That night the consultant on shift looking after Joshua feels that the condition of his lungs has improved sufficiently for him to be 'weaned off' ECMO, allowing him to breathe with his own lungs again. The next morning, Hoa and I go to see Joshua. The weaning has been unsuccessful, but more worrying, he has developed major swelling around his stomach and abdomen. The cause of the swelling isn't clear.

Throughout this time Hoa has been sending messages to her parents in Vietnam. Hoa's mother had booked tickets to visit England the previous month, expecting to come and visit her daughter and to help with her new grandson. A few days earlier my parents had driven to Newcastle bringing our daughter Emily with them, staying in a nearby hotel.

Over the next 24 hours things become clearer. Joshua's left lung is more severely damaged by the infection than was previously realised. During the weaning process his left lung starts to bleed from an area that had become necrotic – cells in the lung tissue had died. His situation then becomes ever more desperate. A drain inserted into his abdomen releases a large amount of blood, but the bleeding is profuse and unstoppable, the situation made so much worse by the blood-thinning Heptin needed to stop blood clots in the ECMO equipment.

The staff try hard to save Joshua. In desperate measures, the Heptin is stopped and a second ECMO machine put on standby to allow a quick changeover should any blood clots occur in the system.

There will be one final chance to save him.

On the night of November 4th the staff make a final attempt to wean Joshua off the ECMO machine. If successful and Joshua is able to sustain breathing with his own lungs, an operation on the necrotic part of Joshua's lung can be performed and Joshua would be likely to survive. We stay with Joshua as long as we can that evening before going to our flat for the night. We know that the next few hours are critical. We don't sleep and, although I'm not religious, we both pray that Joshua will make it through.

In the early hours of the next morning I phone the Unit. Joshua is still being weaned. He is almost 100% off the ECMO machine and things are looking good. I update my parents who meet in the relatives' waiting area of the Unit. We are anxious to see Joshua who we assume must now have been weaned off ECMO. After a while my father and I walk along the corridor and look into the room where Joshua is. Alarmingly, there are a large number of people around Joshua. Noticing us at the window, a consultant we haven't met before comes to the door and tells us, quite abruptly, that the wean was not successful and that Joshua is back on full ECMO.

My father and I break down in tears. We go back into the relatives' room and the whole family cries together. We know that Joshua does not have long left. A few moments later, a male consultant comes into the room, looking sorrowful. Joshua is bleeding profusely. It might be possible to operate to remove the necrotic lung while he is still on ECMO, but to do so would be futile and only serve to extend Joshua's suffering.

We simply can't cope anymore and, in tears, agree to let Joshua go. I beg the doctor to help Joshua go without any pain and he nods his head and assures me he will. At exactly 12.15pm he comes back into the room and tells us that Joshua has gone.

I have never felt such pain or grief, but worse still is seeing the pain in my wife. The emptiness and sorrow on her face is unbearable. The staff at the Freeman Hospital are kind and caring. They tell us that Joshua will be stitched up and we can then say our final goodbyes and hold him for the last time. A short while later we go into the room. We let Emily come with us; this is her brother and we want the family to be together. This was the first time we have seen Joshua without the tubes, wires, patches and the rest of the equipment that surrounded him since the day after his birth. He is lying on the bed in a nappy. His skin is more yellow than normal and there is a small drop of blood from a cannula that had been in his arm. He has stitches in his abdomen where the drain for his lung had been. Most of all, he looks like a perfect and beautiful baby boy.

We take it in turns to hold him, kiss him, tell him how much we love him and how sorry we are. And then we have to say goodbye. In the nicest possible way, the nurses tell us that Joshua has to be moved out of the room and we understand. Other babies need to be cared for and staff need to do their best and carry on with their jobs. We talk about the practicalities - where Joshua's body would be sent. We are given the option of taking Joshua's body away with us back to Cumbria by car. This we simply can't face; Joshua is taken to the mortuary.

Before we leave the hospital my father and I have a brief conversation with the consultant. He explains that he has notified the Coroner of the circumstances of Joshua's death. We are told that because the cause of death is not in dispute, a post-mortem is not necessary and the Coroner will not open an inquest. However, the consultant says that if we were to raise a complaint about Joshua's care at FGH he would expect it to be taken very seriously. None of this really sinks in at the time and we leave the Unit.

We decide to spend a night at the hotel where my parents are staying and drive back home the following day. It is a cold

November evening. The smell of fireworks is in the air and we hear the occasional crackle and bang as we walk to the flat to fetch our things.

We get to the hotel later that evening. The night is spent in tears, desolate and empty. The next day my parents take Emily in their car. It takes some time to get Hoa into our car. She doesn't want to move. On the way back home Hoa tries to jump out of the moving car twice. Each time I have to swerve and stop violently.

My wife simply doesn't want to live. Our lives will never be the same again.

Eventually, later that day, we arrive home. Emily stays with my mum and dad that night. We need some time alone. Opening the door to the house we walk over the post lying on the doormat. It's a mixture of 'congratulations' and 'condolence' cards. We can't do anything but sit and cry together.

The next few days go by in a blur. I tell the neighbours what has happened. All the practical things that need to be done are done. Joshua's body is still in Newcastle. We visit the local Dalton undertaker, a wonderfully kind and compassionate man. He helps us make arrangements for Joshua's body to be transferred. He tells us that they will arrange the funeral free of charge. My sister and brother-in-law travel from their home in Yorkshire to visit us on the day that Joshua's body arrives. We all visit Joshua together.

Seeing Joshua is hard. He still looks like the perfect baby boy we held in our arms just two weeks before, but his skin is yellow and he is cold and stiff. His eyes are closed. I take some comfort from the fact that he seems at peace.

A day later, Hoa's mum arrives from Vietnam. We pick her up from Manchester airport, passing the undertakers on our way home. She says that she wants to see Joshua straight away. Her visit has been planned in advance and was intended to be a joyful one. She is supposed to be helping us to look after her new grandson, just as she cared for his newborn sister just a few years before.

Despite the tears and the distress, the arrival of Hoa's mum is a big relief. I know how much Hoa needs her comfort and support.

In those early days nothing makes much sense to us. We get through each day as best we can. We choose a coffin and arrange a day for the funeral. Hoa and I visit Joshua for the last time. We write him a note on the back of a photo of Hoa, Emily and me, which says how much we love him and, putting a soft toy elephant next to him, we say our final goodbye. We choose the words for his headstone: *Our little fighter, always remembered.*

The funeral is the next day. It is a beautifully sunny day and Joshua is laid to rest in the cemetery next to a small row of other babies' memorials. We stand with our friends and relatives around the grave as we say our goodbyes. Hoa's mum is inconsolable.

Before the funeral I walk into town to the local florist to buy flowers for the grave. The lady behind the counter asks if the flowers are for someone special; I explain the circumstances and she starts to cry. She tells me that in 2004 she had lost a baby girl who was also buried in Dalton cemetery. She says that in the case of her daughter, 'it was just one of those things' and 'there was nothing anyone could have done'.

Little do I realise the significance of that conversation.

We will never forget the funeral. Our friends and neighbours all come including our community midwife, who was on holiday when Joshua was born. We have a small wake afterwards at the nearby house of my parents. The love, support and comfort we are shown is huge. The days after are very hard; nights are spent in tears, taking down the cot and packing away the baby clothes we'd excitedly bought a few weeks before. It is a time of huge grief and pain.

But my determination to find out what really happened to Joshua begins to grow. I need answers about what happened to my baby son; no other parents should ever lose a baby the way we lost Joshua. My focus starts to shift from grief towards the need to find out the truth.

Chapter 2 - Hope and despair

You can never really get over the death of a child; it will remain with you forever. All you can do is build your life around it. As the first huge waves of grief subsided and I began to collect my thoughts, I knew I had to find out what had happened to Joshua. Little did I know just what a long and arduous journey I had begun.

After the funeral I went back to the chronology notes that we had made while Joshua was on ECMO in Newcastle. I typed them up and added some of the questions that were beginning to form in my mind. It became the document that, on November 14th, my father and I hand-delivered to the Chief Executive's office at Furness General Hospital. The final paragraph read:

I believe that if Joshua and my wife had been given the correct treatment at Furness General, our son would still be with us. It is clear to me that many serious mistakes were made during the critical days of labour and the first 24 hours of his life in the care of Furness General Hospital.

I also wrote to John Hutton, our local Member of Parliament and to Tim Farron, the MP for Westmorland and Lonsdale, whose constituency was served by the Morecambe Bay Trust.

Letter writing was something I was going to have to get used to.

My letter to John Hutton concluded:

We are now mourning the loss of our son. I will never understand why he was so neglected during his first 24 hours at FGH.

I am asking you to ensure that a full and comprehensive inquiry takes place into the circumstances at FGH that led to the death of my baby son. It is vital that this should include a wide-ranging review of the management of maternity services at this hospital as well as the specific treatment of our child.

Please inform me as soon as possible of the steps that you feel able to take to ensure that this matter is fully investigated.

A few days later I had a phone call from the Customer Services Manager at University Hospitals of Morecambe Bay Trust, suggesting that my wife and I should meet with the Head of Midwifery and the Maternity Risk Manager. We considered this but decided against it. Before any meeting, we needed to have written answers to the questions we had asked.

On Friday November 21st I contacted the Customer Services Manager and asked for copies of the medical records relating to the care received at FGH by Joshua and my wife. I needed this information to make sense of what had happened and I assumed that at least some of it must be contained in the medical records.

A few days later I received a phone call from the Trust telling me that copies of the medical records would be available to collect that afternoon.

Just before I was about to collect them I received another phone call with news that I couldn't quite believe: the

Customer Services Manager told me the records were ready, but that a document had 'gone missing'. I asked what document, and she replied, 'Joshua's observation chart'.

I was shocked. How could such a vital record have 'gone missing'? Why were we only finding out about it now, on November 25th? Joshua had died nearly three weeks ago and it was four weeks after he first collapsed while in the care of Furness General Hospital. Why had it taken so long for the Trust to discover that vital medical records had 'gone missing'? What had the Trust been doing during this period? If the records could not be found at that time, why wasn't this fact immediately noted? Had the Trust carried out any investigation into how they had gone 'missing'? Could they have been deliberately destroyed?

The Customer Services Manager attempted to reassure me, explaining that any observations recorded on the chart would also have been written down in other records. My concerns would turn out to be fully justified. I remembered that Hoa had actually seen the vital document - a yellow sheet of paper. She had even remembered some of Joshua's temperatures recorded on it. This was to be a key fact in the investigations that followed.

Later that day my father and I collected the records and my worst fears were realised. Not only was the observation chart missing but virtually no records of any of Joshua's observations existed at all, from the time he was transferred to the postnatal ward to the moment of his collapse.

Later that day I wrote more letters to the Chief Executive and the MPs John Hutton and Tim Farron.

Not long after I was contacted again. This time we were told that the Chief Executive of the Trust, Tony Halsall, wanted to visit us at our home to talk about the Trust's response to Joshua's death.

The meeting took place on November 27th. My father and mother joined us. Why was the Chief Executive coming to see us? Was he demonstrating his genuine concern or were there other motives?

Halsall arrived along with the Customer Services Manager and another manager from the Children's and Family Services Division of the Trust.

We talked through in detail the sequence of events that preceded Joshua's death and went over the questions. Halsall seemed sincere, upset and genuinely shocked by what we told him. The part of the story that I just couldn't understand was that we had repeatedly raised concerns about Joshua's condition and asked if he needed antibiotics but were reassured, adamantly, that he was fine. How could this have happened? I asked Halsall if other similar incidents had happened at the Maternity Unit. There followed an uncomfortable pause. The Customer Services Manager looked sheepish. Eventually Halsall answered: 'Of course, other babies will have sadly died. But nothing like this has happened before and the Unit has a very safe record'.

Halsall then asked me 'what I wanted' - a very odd question. I told him we wanted the full truth regarding what happened to our son and to make sure that nothing like it would ever happen again.

Before the meeting concluded, Halsall told us that he would speak to the Medical Director of the Trust, who would ensure that Joshua's death was investigated as a Serious Untoward Incident (SUI). We did not fully understand the significance of this at the time. A SUI is the formal designation in the

NHS that is applied when something has gone seriously wrong. It is supposed to trigger a standard system of formal investigation.

I explained that we were particularly concerned about the missing observation chart and, in response, we were assured that an independent review would establish what had happened and we would be given a chance to meet the investigating team.

A few days later we received a letter from the Trust telling us that two external independent experts would be carrying out a review of the circumstances of Joshua's death. These experts would also want to meet my wife and I to go through our chronology of events. This meeting was set for December 31st, 2008 – New Year's Eve.

It seemed like we had done all we could at this point. We would have to wait to hear back from the Trust but at least a process was underway which should give us answers.

The following days and weeks were full of despair. It is hard to explain the emptiness and grief. I was numb. I became incapable of thinking about anything other than the moments of Joshua's life, which I relived again and again. Then there were the feelings of guilt: if only I'd been more assertive about the need for antibiotics. Should I have insisted Joshua was seen by a doctor? If I had, surely his death could have been avoided. I was not alone in feeling guilty. My mother told me that she felt the same. She said she was worried about Joshua when she held him during the few hours that my parents joined us at the hospital. My dad has told me that she still feels this sense of guilt years later.

Worst of all was seeing the pain and despair in my wife. Hoa spent most of each day crying with grief. She had to deal with things that no mother should ever have to experience. While Joshua was alive in Newcastle she had been able to express milk, which was given to him via a tube into his stomach. In the days following Joshua's death Hoa was given medication to stop the production of milk, but this took time to take effect. Seeing her pain in having to express milk that should have been for Joshua, only to be thrown away, was heartbreaking and somehow deeply symbolic of the cruelty of the situation. Neither of us could sleep well. My sleep was interrupted with vivid dreams and waking up crying or shouting for someone to help, only to realise it was all too late.

I'm not someone who is usually emotionally dependent, but in those early days I looked for all the help I could find. I thought about Joshua's death night and day. I was becoming very difficult to live with.

I made contact with the charity Sands (the Stillbirth and Neonatal Death charity) and we spoke at length with one of their helpline staff. It was hugely helpful to talk about Joshua and what we were going through with someone who listened and understood. I also found out that Sands had a web forum for bereaved parents so I registered and tentatively explored the forum postings. Some posts were specific questions, but often the posts were expressions of feelings and emotions or simply people telling their stories. Reading the posts was both sad and helpful; we weren't alone in our grief, many others had experienced what we were going through. The forum opened my eyes to just how many others had also lost a baby. I eventually posted Joshua's story and the Sands forum became a valued source of advice, comfort and support.

On December 9th, 2008 I decided to write to both the Coroner in Newcastle and our local Coroner in Cumbria to ask if they would consider opening an inquest. The local Coroner, Ian Smith, responded very quickly but only to say that the decision as to whether an inquest could be opened rested with the Newcastle Coroner alone. On December 15th the Newcastle Coroner, David Mitford, responded. His letter stated:

Although you have now raised a variety of concerns... They are matters which, if you wish to pursue them, could be the subject of an appropriate complaint to the hospitals involved who will have complaints procedures to deal with this sort of situation.

It seemed very unlikely we would be able to persuade Mr Mitford to open an inquest.

In the following weeks we started to put together a plan towards regaining some sort of normality. Although I'm not religious, Hoa and I talked in spiritual terms about Joshua. We told each other that Joshua knew how much we loved and missed him and that if we had another child, it would be as if Joshua's spirit would come back to us. These thoughts, however irrational, were part of our way of coping. Hoa was brought up as a Buddhist in Vietnam; she was also trying to cope in her own way even though I did not fully understand it. During this period our common grief brought us closer together.

In mid-December I decided I was ready to go back to work. I was working in the nuclear industry, at Sellafield on the Cumbrian Coast, and my employer was very generous and understanding. I had been off work for more than a month, but I could not have returned before. At first I felt disconnected and distant, then slowly a sense of normality returned. My work colleagues reacted in different ways. One or two spoke to me about what had happened and offered support, but others didn't acknowledge our loss at all. Maybe they were frightened of causing upset or simply did not know what to say.

Re-establishing a routine was helpful for both of us. Throughout all of this we had Emily, our wonderful daughter who was approaching four and who provided us with comfort and purpose. Our parents were also strongly supportive, especially for Emily who had also been through a traumatic experience.

Hoa and I joined a local gym. Keeping busy and getting exercise helped distract from our heartache. I began to count the days to the meeting with the promised 'investigation team'.

Two medical experts, a Senior Midwife and an Obstetrician from another Trust, together with a note taker, arrived in the early evening of December 31st, 2008. My mum and dad joined us. The two experts had statements taken from staff in relation to Joshua's death although it was very clear they had no intention of sharing these with us.

We went through the events. Given our concerns about the missing observation chart, Hoa recounted her recollection of what she remembered about Joshua, including recalling two specific temperatures she saw on the observation chart. These were 35.8° and 36.1°.

Following this, we then asked the following question, which has since turned out to be of vital importance.

Given the fact that Joshua's critical medial records have 'gone missing', were the events that my wife and I have just described fully consistent with the statements that staff have provided in response to your investigation?

We received an unequivocal assurance that there were no discrepancies and that staff had reported exactly the same events as we had.

This came as a great relief. If the staff involved in Joshua's care had reported the same events as Hoa and I, the significance of the gaps in Joshua's medical records and the missing observation chart seemed less important. At this stage, despite the loss of records, we were confident that the Trust really were committed to establishing the full truth and that any necessary learning would take place. I needed to secure this reassurance before I would be able to fully come to terms with what had happened and move on from our loss. This was going to be far harder than I could ever have imagined.

In early January 2009 we had some important news - Hoa was pregnant. Of all places, we found out at the gym. We had bought a pregnancy test on the way - really just a spontaneous purchase. Neither of us thought Hoa would be pregnant. But she was. We sat in the gym foyer, both in tears, and attracted some strange looks. The mix of emotions was hard to explain: joy, happiness, guilt and sadness. Most of all I realised this news would give us some hope for the future, a reason to be strong and a way to move forward. However irrational, we couldn't help feeling that perhaps this was a way for Joshua to come back to us. While my rational mind completely rejected any notion that this could be true, we talked about and took some comfort from these thoughts.

Over the following weeks I kept in regular contact with the Trust, mainly through the Customer Services Manager, chasing progress on the investigation and seeking reassurances that our concerns were being addressed.

I also started to research more about what happened to Joshua. I Googled papers on neonatal sepsis and found out that the most common neonatal infection was called Group B Streptococcus (GBS), but that Joshua had Streptococcal Pneumonia (also called Pneumococcus), which was much rarer. It is a more aggressive type of infection associated with higher neonatal mortality. Pre-labour Rupture of Membranes (PROM) was a key risk.

Pneumococcus, while being a rare infection in a neonate, was common in adults and was associated with sore throats and headaches, exactly what my wife and I had been suffering from in the days before Joshua's birth. In terms of signs of infection in a neonate, while these can include a raised temperature, a more common indication was a low temperature or difficulty in maintaining a normal temperature. A baby who was lethargic, mucousy or reluctant to feed, all pointed to possible infection.

The more I read, the more I realised that Joshua had been showing clear signs of infection before his collapse at Furness General. I went over and over the events in my mind and, although I told myself that it wasn't my fault, my feelings of personal guilt continued to haunt me. If only I had done more to help Joshua when he still had a chance. The more I read, the more determined I became to seek answers to how and why Joshua's death happened.

I made contact with an organisation called Action against Medical Accidents (AvMA) which provided advice and information, but the next steps all depended on the Trust's investigation report.

In early February I was contacted by the Customer Services Manager and a date was set to meet Halsall who would hand us the investigation report. My anxiety began to build.

None of the medical records I had seen gave a clear indication of what had happened to Joshua. We had a real fear that the report would be a whitewash and would deny responsibility.

When the day arrived Hoa, my mum and dad and I went together to Furness General. We arrived before Halsall and waited for him. It's strange the little details you remember, but I recall that Halsall looked flustered and had a cut on his chin from shaving. We were led into a small room and all sat around the table. Halsall told us the report clearly acknowledged that Joshua had been failed and that as a consequence, he had lost his fight for life. He told us that on behalf of himself and the Trust, they were deeply sorry. While the Trust couldn't do anything to change what had happened to Joshua, they would do everything they could to make sure it wouldn't happen again.

We were tearful, but thanked Halsall for what he had said. We were then handed the report itself. My first thought was that it was incredibly thin. Taking out the title and contents page, it was just seven pages long. This report was to be the first of many.

The conclusions were as follows:

1) *There was a failure to monitor for or recognise multiple signs of possible neonatal sepsis. As a consequence antibiotics were started later than they could have been which may have contributed to the eventual tragic outcome in the case.*

2) *The most effective way of preventing sepsis in a neonate following pre labour rupture of membranes is to start antibiotics prior to delivery. However, this is only routinely recommended when the membranes rupture prior to 37 weeks or if the mother is pyrexial in labour. Staff at Furness General should not be criticised for not starting antibiotics prior to delivery because, by their estimation,*

based on NICE recommended practice the membranes did
not rupture until after 37 weeks.

There were 6 recommendations.

1) *The Trust should review and clarify its policy for the management of pre-labour rupture of membranes.*

2) *The Trust should review and enhance its policies for the monitoring and care of neonates including clear indications for medical review by a neonatal paediatrician.*

3) *The Trust should provide training for staff in relation to the care of the neonate and in particular sign of sepsis.*

4) *The temperature in the rooms in which neonates are nursed should be monitored on a continuous basis.*

5) *The general standard of record keeping needs to be improved and should be subject to regular audit.*

6) *Handover of care requires better documentation and clarity as to who is the named carer at all times.*

Our initial reaction was a sense of relief. We had a clear acceptance that Joshua had been failed. However, the report also appeared to leave a large number of issues unaddressed.

The report noted that three midwives had written in their statements that a paediatrician had been contacted in relation to Joshua and advice had been received to monitor him, but none of the paediatricians on duty remembered taking such a call. The report simply left this issue unresolved.

It stated:

Of particular note there is no mention in the records of Mrs Titcombe being unwell in the days prior to delivery although Mr and Mrs Titcombe clearly remember telling the midwives about this.

My wife and I had had detailed discussions with staff about not feeling well before the birth. We had a very clear recollection of this. It was not possible that this was something that the staff could 'misremember'.

Mrs Titcombe advised at one stage that Joshua was in the heated cot with an overhead heater over him as well, in an effort to raise his temperature.

The report recognised 'This would be outside normal practice' but the authors did not make it clear whether they accepted that this had happened or not. This brought to mind the statements made at the meeting at our house on December 31st, when we were assured that the statements of the FGH staff were fully consistent with our chronology.

I had other concerns. The report was undated and not signed by anyone. There were no page numbers. The formatting was poor and some sentences suddenly cut off part way through, as if the report had been hastily edited. It felt like a document that had been written over a few hours, not something that had taken three months to write relating to the preventable death of a child.

At the time of these events I had been working as Project Manager on a large nuclear development at Sellafield. I had received regular training about safety procedures in the nuclear industry. At Sellafield an investigation into a rusty bolt would be more detailed and professionally presented than this report.

I raised with Halsall the fact that the reported recommendations seem very general. What were the recommendations and actions in relation to the actions of individual midwives? He told us that the recommendations in relation to individual staff would be addressed through a different process – a system known as 'midwifery supervision'. There was a body called the Local Supervising Authority (LSA), who would be carrying out an investigation to produce another report into Joshua's care that would address any failures of care and actions needed in relation to individual midwives. The LSA and system of midwifery supervision in place at the Trust at the time would prove to play a huge part in the events that followed.

We had mixed feelings after this meeting. Our first fears that the Trust might deny outright any responsibility for what happened to Joshua were laid to rest. We were very relieved about that. The Trust had accepted that Joshua had died because of clear failures of care for which the Trust had accepted responsibility.

However, this still left large gaps. I wanted much more detail in relation to specific failures and whether these were systemic or just unfortunate errors of judgement.

I began to have doubts about the statements that had been given to the inquiry team by the midwives. Why had we not been allowed to see these statements?

Chapter 3 - Searching for answers

Over the next week I thought about the report a lot. I decided I would write a detailed letter to my MP, John Hutton, setting out what I saw as clear management failings. The Trust's report alluded to the fact that the unit was understaffed. Why had this happened? Why were systems for handover of care so inadequate? Why were the staff looking after Joshua not trained to recognise basic signs of sepsis?

I also asked questions about the missing observation chart and the fact that none of the paediatricians on duty had admitted to receiving a call about Joshua. I wanted to ensure that the individual accountabilities associated with what happened to Joshua were properly investigated. I sent this letter to Hutton with a courtesy copy to Halsall on February 20th, 2009. A few days later Halsall replied, stating that we would receive a full response to the letter.

Around the same time I started to research more about how serious safety incidents in the NHS were managed. In my professional life I was familiar with Health and Safety legislation, particularly the Health and Safety and Work Act (HSWA) 1974. I had been on a number of training courses in managing safety and I understood the regulatory framework within which the Health and Safety Executive operated.

The piece of legislation that underpinned the whole ethos and culture in which I was used to working was Section 3 of the HSWA. In simple terms, this places a duty on every employer to take all 'reasonably practicable' steps not to expose people to risks to their health and safety. In the construction industry this requirement is taken extremely seriously - a core requirement before carrying out any work activity on a construction site would be to write a Work Safety Plan and carry out a Risk Assessment. These documents would detail each step of the work activity and highlight any potential health and safety risks. The process would ensure that any identified risks were appropriately documented and work would only be authorised to proceed if these documents were signed and approved by a safety professional. In my professional career there had always been huge emphasis on safety. Nothing was more important.

The circumstances of Joshua's death made me think about how the culture of safety I was used to at work was so different from what had happened to Joshua. In my working life a simple task like putting up a ladder to work from an elevated position would require the risks to be thought about, controlled and documented. Joshua was a baby who was recognised to be at risk by the midwives that were responsible for his care. Yet the possible risks to Joshua didn't seem to have been thought about at all.

The Trust's investigation report had noted that 'three midwives had written in their statements that a paediatrician had been contacted in relation to Joshua and advice had been received to monitor him and place him under observation', yet the Trust stated that the staff who were responsible for monitoring Joshua were not trained in the basic signs of neonatal sepsis.

I had read that around 1 in every 100[1] babies develop a neonatal infection after birth. If staff designated to monitor babies thought to be at risk of infection weren't trained to recognise the signs, wasn't it just a matter of time before a tragedy like Joshua's death happened? Did the Trust have a HSWA duty to take 'reasonably practicable' steps not to expose babies like Joshua to risks like this?

If so, if they failed in this HSWA duty, who would investigate and what action would be taken?

I subsequently made contact with the Health and Safety Executive by email and was assured that they were looking carefully at the circumstances of what had happened to Joshua and would write to inform me what action they would take in due course. This was to be only the start of my correspondence with the HSE, who would go on to state repeatedly that the issues associated with Joshua's death were outside their remit to investigate.

I also read about the Nursing and Midwifery Council (NMC). All nurses and midwives practising in the UK must be registered by the NMC. The NMC website explained that the NMC has a responsibility to protect the public by ensuring that all registrants are fit to practice. I prepared a PowerPoint presentation which explained what happened to Joshua and sent this, along with a letter setting out my concerns about his care, to the NMC.

Over the next few weeks, with Hoa's pregnancy progressing, we also spent a lot of time thinking about the new baby and

---

[1] http://www.ncbi.nlm.nih.gov/pubmed/20876594 'With the inclusion of coagulase negative Staphylococci (CoNS), the incidence of all neonatal infection was 8/1000 live births and 71/1000 neonatal admissions (2007-2008).'

where we would have it. There was no way we wanted to go back to Furness General. However, the alternatives were not obvious. There were two other Maternity Units in the area: a midwifery led unit in Kendal, which was around 40 minutes away by road, and a consultant led unit in Lancaster. The latter was around an hour's drive away, but possibly more depending on traffic and A590 obstructions, which are common. Joshua was born very quickly so we were concerned about these journey times. We therefore started to think about the possibility of a home birth and this option began to seem like the best way forward.

On March 25th we received a response from Halsall to our letter. While it did not address all our concerns it did seem like an honest effort. It stated that if Joshua had also received antibiotics at the same time my wife was given them he would have had a 90% chance of survival. He also promised that the Trust would engage an external consultant to carry out a management review of the Maternity Unit at FGH. In terms of the individual accountabilities of staff involved in Joshua's care, Halsall repeated that the Local Supervising Authority would address these issues as part of their investigation. He also stated that the Trust had contacted the NHS Litigation Authority about arranging compensation for Joshua's death. This wasn't something that my family and I were prioritising, but if it could be managed without involving solicitors it was certainly something we welcomed.

In the following weeks I thought a great deal about the situation we were in and discussed the issues with Hoa and my mum and dad. We all felt that Halsall had tried to ensure that lessons were being learned from Joshua's death and his interactions with us had been sincere and genuine. At the same time, there remained some big issues and unanswered questions that I still couldn't put out of my mind.

Was it really possible that Joshua's observation chart had been innocently lost? How was it possible that three midwives recalled that a paediatrician had been phoned in relation to Joshua, yet none of the paediatricians on duty at the time would admit to taking the call? While the Trust had assured us that the midwifery staff had all reported the same sequence of events as my wife and I, how could we know if this was true given the lack of documentation and the lack of detail in the Trust's report? How had the management of the Unit allowed the situation to get so bad that the sequence of events that led to Joshua's death was possible in the first place? What changes were needed to make sure nothing like this happened again?

These thoughts went around and around in my mind. The scale of failures that had occurred were simply too important to walk away from. Despite feeling largely positive about how Halsall had responded up until that point, I decided that the right thing to do was to push for an independent review that addressed these issues.

At the time the NHS regulatory system and complaints process were going through major changes. The regulator of the NHS was then the Healthcare Commission (HCC). The HCC also acted as a second tier for complaints made about the NHS. This meant that if patients or families weren't happy with the response they had received from a hospital or Trust they could refer their complaint to the HCC to investigate. The final stage of the complaints process was through referral to the Parliamentary and Health Service Ombudsman (PHSO). This meant that if a patient or member of their family remained unhappy after going to the HCC they could make a referral to the PHSO who would be the final arbitrator on the complaint. However, this system was about to be fundamentally changed.

From April 1st, 2009 the HCC ceased to exist and was replaced by a new organisation called the Care Quality Commission (CQC). The CQC would no longer also act as the second tier of the complaints process and instead patients or families unhappy with a local response to a complaint could now only refer the matter to the Ombudsman.

On April 4th, 2009 I wrote to the Ombudsman requesting an investigation into the outstanding concerns I had about what happened to Joshua. Although I didn't know it at the time we were, in fact, guinea pigs entering a new and untried system.

I also wrote to the Trust asking for copies of all the statements prepared by staff which had been used by the investigators. I wanted to confirm that the staff had indeed reported the same events that my wife and I had detailed in our chronology we had submitted to the Trust shortly after Joshua's death. We had previously been reassured that our chronology had been accepted by the investigators and was not disputed by the Trust or any of the staff involved in Joshua's care. I was sure that being provided with copies of the statements made by the midwives would be straightforward.

Around this time I also started to clarify in my mind how best we could achieve what we wanted for Joshua. This was the complete truth to ensure that lasting lessons were learned from his death and that all the actions necessary to prevent such a tragic loss of life would be fully implemented. We wanted no more avoidable deaths.

I had become friendly with a reporter from the local paper. She had personal experience of losing a baby. I told her about Joshua's story and agreed to let the paper cover it. I trusted her to be sensitive and balanced. I wanted her piece to reflect what had happened and that Joshua's death was preventable, emphasising that, although the Trust had responded responsibly, important questions remained unanswered. We therefore wanted the Ombudsman to investigate.

On Saturday April 18th, 2009 the local paper covered the story on the front page. There was a big response to the piece with many supportive comments left on the newspaper website. There were also comments from people that mentioned their own poor experiences of care at the same Maternity Unit.

The next day my wife and I took Emily for a walk and we stopped at a local play area. While sitting on a bench watching Emily play, I had a chance conversation with a lady who proceeded to tell me about her experience at FGH. Her story shocked me. She described a situation that sounded very similar to what happened to Joshua involving her baby boy, born just a few weeks before Joshua. Her baby had survived, but what she told me about trying to raise concerns with staff and not being listened to felt all too familiar. This conversation, together with comments I'd seen on-line following the local press report, led me to question whether Joshua's death really was an isolated failure or part of a much more significant pattern of safety failures at the Maternity Unit around the time Joshua was born.

Over the next few weeks I wrote to a number of different organisations. I wrote to the police, hand delivering the letter and supporting documents to the local police station, asking for the circumstances of Joshua's missing observation chart to be investigated. I also wrote to the newly formed regulator, the Care Quality Commission, and provided them with as much information about Joshua's death as possible. In addition, I had also learned that Morecambe Bay was an aspiring Foundation Trust – which would give them a much higher degree of independence from the Strategic Health Authority and the Department of Health - and were in the process of being assessed by another regulator called Monitor. I did not then know much about the structure of NHS hospital services or Foundation Trusts, and nothing at all about Monitor, but I found out as much as I could through research on the internet.

I soon started to get responses. The Ombudsman assigned a case officer to our complaint. The HSE wrote to say that they didn't investigate issues involving clinical judgements, but would be carrying out some work looking at management standards within the Trust. The police responded to say that an officer had been to see Halsall. I received a written response indicating that the police believed that there was no evidence that anyone had deliberately destroyed the missing records and that their view was that everyone involved had been open and honest about what happened to Joshua. Despite my protests and the exchange of a number of emails, the senior officer involved made it very clear to me that the Cumbria Police would not be taking any further action.

On the April 24th the Trust responded to my request for copies of the statements from Trust staff by, to my shock, refusing to provide them. They stated that this request was not covered by the Freedom of Information Act (FOI) and that, as they were therefore not legally required to provide them, they were declining to do so.

At that time I understood little about FOI and nothing about the Data Protection Act (DPA). I did not realise that the Trust had a clear legal duty of disclosure of personally relevant documents under DPA, not FOI. But they must have known that.

This was the point when my attitude towards Halsall and the Trust began to change.

Up until then I had genuinely thought that Halsall and the Trust were being honest with me, but this refusal to disclose the midwives' statements prevented me from checking that they really did accept the facts of our chronology. Why would the Trust refuse to provide the statements if there was nothing to hide?

If they were so determined to keep vital facts and records from me then I would be even more determined to get to the truth.

Chapter 4 - Closing ranks

Over the next few weeks I had several email exchanges with the Trust. I was furious they were refusing to share the staff statements with me but nothing I said was making any difference. I also got in touch with the person in charge of the Local Supervising Authority (LSA) investigation. It had been explained to me that the LSA would address the outstanding issues about Joshua's care that the Trust's investigation didn't cover, including looking at the individual actions of the staff involved. This investigation was therefore hugely important. I waited anxiously for the outcome.

I made sure that all the information I had was shared. I was assured that the LSA report would address all the concerns we had about the midwifery care Joshua received.

On June 1st, 2009 I was emailed a copy of the LSA report. I was at work at the time and so I waited until my lunch break to read it. As I read the first few pages my heart sank.

It was a complete whitewash.

I skimmed through the pages. A section entitled, *The management of the fluctuations in the temperature of a high risk baby* read as follows:

The staff were asked for their recollections and any observations they could remember, until the chart could be retrieved from Manchester... This information suggested that the fluctuations in Joshua's temperature were between 36.4°C and 36.8°C, which did not prompt a request for a paediatric review of this baby with an additional risk factor (Hoa's pyrexia), but was managed by warming a cold room and the use of a cot warmer.

It continued:

Further investigation by the Head of Midwifery revealed that this degree of fluctuation in a newborn's temperature may not have prompted a request for a paediatric review by other midwives in the service either, but may have been seen as the normal variation in temperature of a newborn that can occur in response to the environment.

I could not believe what I was reading.

Hoa clearly recalled seeing a temperature on Joshua's observation chart of 35.8°. When we met the external experts who carried out the Trust's review we gave them this information and we were reassured that the Trust had accepted this and that nothing we had said conflicted with the midwives' statements. To say that Joshua's temperatures varied between 36.4° and 36.8° simply wasn't true. Of course, my mind jumped to the fact that the observation chart where my wife had observed records of lower temperatures had 'gone missing'.

As I read more, things only got worse. The report included answers to some specific questions I had raised. In relation to Hoa feeling poorly before the birth and telling staff on the first visit that she had a headache and sore throat, the report read:

Midwives A and B have no recollection of a sore throat being reported to them...The normal process for the management of women who complain of symptoms not relating to the pregnancy would be referral to the SHO [Senior House Officer] for review. All the midwives have been interviewed and they do not recollect symptoms of a sore throat being reported.

How was this possible? I was with Hoa when we first attended Furness General on the evening her waters broke. She was very distressed and we had a detailed and clear conversation with the staff about how we had both been feeling poorly in the previous few days. I clearly remembered a midwife saying that the illness we described was 'probably a virus' and that there was 'a lot going around'.

There was more. The report stated that the overhead heater, which we knew was placed directly over Joshua (he was heated until at one point his skin was hot to the touch), was simply brought into the room and was not placed directly above Joshua. I knew this wasn't true.

The report drew attention to unresolved discrepancies. A Section entitled, *The lack of a paediatric review of a high risk baby*, stated the following:

Interviews with Midwife E and Midwife F and the midwife in charge, confirm that the Paediatrician was bleeped and informed of the gestation, the prolonged rupture of membranes and the maternal condition. He advised that Joshua should be observed, however these details are not documented in the records. Midwife F has stated that it was a male paediatric doctor who responded to the bleep, but she did not obtain his name. Midwife F and the switchboard logs verify that the paediatric SHO was bleeped and appears to have responded to the call from the Special Care Baby Unit. However, the doctors identified on the paediatric rota, a female SHO and a male middle grade, have been interviewed and deny responding to the call. It is unclear at the time of writing this report what further action is to be undertaken.

It was later revealed that the switchboard logs did *not* verify that a paediatric SHO had been bleeped in relation to Joshua. So this statement was false.

The report appeared to blame the paediatricians for any confusion:

Midwives are concerned that the Paediatric Service has not addressed the issues regarding the paediatric response to the initial management of baby Joshua. If lessons are to be learned there has to be an acknowledgement of their responsibilities and a commitment to ensuring a robust guideline is in place that the Midwifery and Paediatric staff will follow.

The report concluded:

The review of this very sad case has identified potential opportunities for intervention that in this instance were missed, although the changes in Joshua's condition were subtle and as this report suggests - not easily recognised by the midwives. It is impossible to say whether these interventions would have altered the outcome.

How could this report say that the changes in Joshua's condition were 'subtle' when my wife, who was poorly and tired, called a bell by the side of her bed at 2am in the morning (just hours before Joshua eventually collapsed) because Joshua was making 'grunting' sounds and was breathing quickly?

How could the report conclude that it is 'impossible to say whether interventions would have altered the outcome' for Joshua, when the Trust had already acknowledged that his chances of survival would have been around 90% had he been treated appropriately with antibiotics after his birth?

48

I sat at my desk feeling worse than I had ever felt at any time in my life.

Images of Joshua flashed through my mind. I thought about the hope I had, the happiness I felt when he was born, the concerns I had for him, the reassurances I was given that he was fine, the agony of finding out he had collapsed, then watching him fight for his life for days while my wife and I desperately hoped he would pull through and his ultimate death in horrific circumstances.

While I knew that nothing could ever change what had happened or bring Joshua back, a cold anger took hold of me. I had never wanted staff involved in Joshua's care to be unfairly punished or disciplined over what happened, but I did want them to be honest. I needed the truth to be told including an honest acceptance of the consequences for Joshua and my family. I was not going to accept this cover-up.

I printed out a copy of the report and, without saying a word to anyone, left the office, got in my car and started to drive towards home. At first I didn't know where I was going to go; perhaps to my mum and dad's or home to Hoa?

But as I drove I knew that I had to go to Furness General. I drove straight to the hospital. With the report in my hand, I walked through the corridors at FGH towards the Maternity Unit. By chance someone was just leaving so the entrance door, usually locked with a key code system, was open. I walked through and went straight to the main desk. Two members of staff were there. I had been crying in the car and in a broken but loud voice, I demanded to see whoever was in charge.

I said that I wanted to talk 'about my son's death and the lies in this report'. Very quickly I was ushered into a side room. I was left for a moment and then two other members of staff entered. I was in tears.

I told them I was outraged by the dishonesty of the staff involved in Joshua's care and I wouldn't allow them to get away with lying about what really happened to my son. I threw the report on the floor, stormed out of the room and drove home.

The next day I had a scheduled meeting with the LSA in Kendal. Hoa had previously told me that she didn't want to attend the meeting as she found talking about what happened to Joshua difficult. She was now heavily pregnant and I was keen to shelter her as much as possible from the distress of the ongoing situation. However, when Hoa read the LSA report that night she insisted she would attend the meeting. She wanted to be there in person to tell the truth about what happened to her son.

The next day I drove to Kendal with Hoa and my dad. The meeting was truly awful. We were introduced to the author of the report who, I was surprised to learn, as well as being the FGH Supervisor of Midwives was also the Risk Manager for the Trust.

At the start of the meeting Hoa, in tears, described what had happened to Joshua and how she clearly recalled seeing temperatures on 35.8° and 36.1° on the now missing observation chart. She explained that she didn't want to be at the meeting. She was pregnant and had to think about her new baby, but she couldn't stand by while people were being dishonest about what happened to Joshua. It made me feel very proud of her, but also deeply angry.

After all that my wife had suffered why was she having to go through this?

The rest of the meeting was deeply unpleasant and uncomfortable. At one point we were told that 'the only thing the midwives did wrong' in relation to Joshua's care was not 'write down what they did'. Fortunately I had made a decision to record the meeting on my mobile phone. I still have this recording.

As we left the meeting we all shared the strong feeling that the people we had just met were really only interested in sweeping what had happened to Joshua under the carpet.

I became more determined that ever to ensure that this wouldn't happen.

In the following days I wrote a detailed letter of complaint to the LSA and more letters to Halsall, Monitor, CQC, the Police, the NMC and the Ombudsman. I now felt that I was not only dealing with a tragic accident but I was also facing a deliberate cover-up. I wasn't at all confident about what these organisations could achieve, but I felt certain that that the Ombudsman, the last resort of NHS complainants, must at least investigate.

Just a few weeks later, something happened that significantly increased my concerns. On July 3rd, 2009 the local paper ran a story on its front page with the headline *Coroner slams Barrow hospital over stillborn baby death*. The report was about the tragic death of baby Alex Davey-Brady, which had happened at Furness General Hospital just months before Joshua had died.

The report read:

A Coroner has criticised Furness General Hospital and said midwives ran the show over doctors in the tragic case of a stillborn baby.

South and East Cumbria Coroner Ian Smith said that rather than one team working together, he pictured two teams operating side by side.

He said: 'I don't believe the doctors integrated, the midwives ran the show. Dr Sur Roy never examined the mother during the day, which I find strange. He was not as actively involved as he should have been'.

[The baby's father] said he felt there was a terrible lack of communication between the doctors and midwives.

I couldn't believe what I was reading. The words 'the midwives ran the show' echoed in my mind. This phrase seemed to perfectly describe what had happened to Joshua.

I remembered that first meeting I had with Halsall in my living room all those months before.

When I asked Halsall if anything like Joshua's death had happened before there had been an awkward pause. He must have known about this case, which had happened just weeks before Joshua was born. How could he have not recognised the similarities?

Joshua was a baby who had been identified as needing to be closely observed following his mother's illness, yet the first time he was seen by a paediatrician was after his mother found him collapsed 24 hours after his birth.

In Joshua's case too, 'the doctors didn't integrate'. The LSA report said that the midwife who spoke to the doctor, in what is a small Maternity Unit, couldn't identify who she spoke to. How could this be true?

All the doctors on duty at the time denied that they had ever taken a call relating to Joshua. What was going on in that

Maternity Unit when Joshua was born? Had other factors contributed to what happened?

The LSA report seemed to point a finger at the role of the doctors. It implied that, if lessons were to be learned, it was the role of the doctors that needed to be examined.

The Coroner in the story in the local paper was clearly suggesting that something was amiss in the relationships between paediatricians and midwives. If such a dysfunction was also a factor in Joshua's death, was this still going on? Were mothers and babies still at risk? Had there been more deaths in the FGH Maternity Unit that I did not know about?

Chapter 5 - A light in the dark

It was now July 2009. Hoa was seven months pregnant. When we found out we were having a baby girl we decided to call her Jessica. We had spent a considerable amount of time thinking about where she would be born, but now we had decided. We had been having regular meetings with our obstetric consultant, a man who was very understanding of our situation. We talked about the options and were strongly advised against having the baby at either Kendal or Lancaster. Both these hospitals were simply too far from our home to be considered. We were also advised against a homebirth: if anything went wrong we wanted medical help to be available straight away. Instead, we were offered a special plan of care at Furness General. We were told that no midwives involved in Joshua's care would be involved, that a doctor would be present during the birth and that, straight away following delivery, Jessica would be transferred immediately to the Special Care Baby Unit (SCBU) where she would be given precautionary antibiotics and closely monitored.

Although we were anxious about this plan we wanted to choose the safest option and, given the additional arrangements in place, we decided to accept the advice from our consultant. We agreed to have the birth at Furness General.

By this stage I had been contacted directly by the National Health Service Litigation Authority (NHSLA). Following the Trust's investigation, and after talking through with me, Halsall had written to the NHSLA confirming that the Trust had accepted liability for Joshua's preventable death. In these circumstances, the amount of compensation the NHSLA pay in relation to the preventable death of a child is pitifully small. We had been offered an amount equivalent to little more than 6 months of my salary at the time. In my correspondence with the NHSLA I made it clear that we had many unresolved issues in relation to Joshua's death that we were still pursuing but, providing our agreement to accept the offer of compensation did not affect any of these processes, we would accept the settlement.

Just a few weeks after I had read the report about the death of baby Alex Davey-Brady in the local paper I received more disturbing information. The Trust finally released the statements that the midwives involved in Joshua's care had written in order to assist the Trust's investigation.

By this stage I knew from the LSA report that the individuals involved hadn't all been truthful, but I was still shocked when I read the statements. They were very brief and lacking in detail. They were dated around December 2008, more than a month after Joshua had died. Given the lack of records documenting Joshua's care and the fact that Joshua's critical observation chart had 'gone missing', why did it take so long for staff to be asked to give statements about what happened? Shouldn't detailed statements have been taken immediately after he collapsed and was transferred from Furness General in a critical condition?

Despite being reassured by the Trust and the external experts that there were no conflicts between what my wife and I had described and what the staff had reported, we now knew for certain that this wasn't true.

None of the statements acknowledged the true temperatures of 35.8° and 36.1° that my wife had seen on the missing observation chart.

In addition, for the first time, the statements contained a description of Joshua's birth:

07.38am: Joshua cried immediately, APGAR score 9 (one point being deducted for blue extremities).

07.40am: Joshua was then placed in his mother's arms and we held her to turn around to a sitting position.

07.43am: His respiration was now irregular and although his limbs were flexed, his muscle tone was not as good as when he was first born. The room was dim and I explained to the Titcombe's that I would take Joshua to the well lit resuscitaire to examine him properly. Joshua was approximate 5 minutes old when I took him to the resuscitaire. I gave him facial oxygen by mask.

07.44am: After about 30 seconds he cried, he went pink all over and his muscle tone was good.

As I read this I actually thought that the midwife who wrote it must have got Joshua's birth confused with another delivery she might have done that day. However, the statement from the other midwife present when Joshua was born described the same events.

This simply wasn't what happened when Joshua was born. I remembered the facts very clearly.

When Joshua was born he was blue, limp, not breathing and not crying. He did not cry immediately. He only cried after he was given oxygen. After the cord was cut Joshua was taken to a small table on the right hand side of my wife's bed. He was still blue, limp and not crying or breathing. I stood over him and watched as the midwife rubbed his chest and encouraged him to breathe. After what must have been at least another minute she told me she would take him out the room to give him oxygen and that I could go with her. I went with the midwife to the room and watched as Joshua was given oxygen. He then started to breathe and let out a loud cry and went pink. I was anxious to go back to Hoa because I knew she would be worried. I remember the midwife saying not to worry because Hoa would have heard the cry.

I couldn't understand why the midwives had described Joshua's birth so differently from what really happened. Was the fact that Joshua was not breathing at birth and required oxygen before breathing for himself important? Later on I learned that Joshua had swallowed a large amount of meconium (this is the substance babies produce with their first bowel movements) whilst he was still in the womb. Did this explain why Joshua struggled and needed oxygen before breathing properly after his birth?

The statements also confirmed other misinformation that we knew had been accepted as true in the LSA report. There was no mention of the discussion my wife and I had with staff at our first visit to Furness General about feeling poorly with sore throats and headaches.

The statements also described the use of the overhead heater, claiming that it was not placed above Joshua but merely placed within the room because the room was cold. We knew this wasn't true. Many of the midwives' statements described the room Joshua was in as being cold yet my wife and I remember the room being very warm. This began to look like a collective fabrication.

The discrepancies and misinformation went on and on. In the following days I prepared a detailed spreadsheet setting out the information in the statements and the conflicts between them and what my wife and I knew to be the truth. I sent copies of this spreadsheet to all the organisations I had been in touch with. I thought that by now the need for a proper external investigation into these events must be obvious and urgent.

Soon after receiving these statements I arranged to meet with a senior detective from Cumbria Police to discuss the growing concerns I had. The initial response from the police regarding the missing records was that this wasn't a significant issue: the staff had been open and honest about the events and there were no discrepancies between what my wife and I recalled and what the staff reported. I now knew for certain that this wasn't true. I also now knew that Joshua's death was not an isolated case and may, in fact, have been a consequence of systematic failures at the Maternity Unit.

On Monday, July 27th I met with Detective Chief Superintendent Iain Goulding at my home. From the outset it was clear to me that this was going to be a very different discussion to those I had previously had with Cumbria Police. DCS Goulding listened carefully to what I had to say and, far from being dismissive, he clearly sympathised with the situation and understood our concerns. He suggested that I contact the Coroner again. Importantly, I was also told that although Cumbria Police would not at the present time open an investigation into Joshua's death, the situation would be kept under review. The role of Cumbria Police would turn out to be crucial.

Later that same day, following DCS Goulding's suggestion, I wrote again to the local Coroner to ask him to consider opening an Inquest. I outlined that although the cause of Joshua's death was not in dispute (uncontrollable bleeding to a necrotic part of his left lung due to pneumococcal infection) we now knew that the statements made by midwives had been seriously falsified and that the key records of his care had been lost. Joshua died because of a lack of appropriate medical intervention, appalling record keeping and what appears to be an unsatisfactory working relationship between doctors and midwives. Far from being a one-off event, there could be unresolved deep rooted issues that present a continuing risk to mothers and babies attending the maternity service at Furness General Hospital.

On the July 31st I received a response from Mr Smith, the local Coroner, which was unhelpful to say the least. His letter stated that I needed to write to the Newcastle Coroner, not him, but went on to say:

I can only think that recent publicity about other deaths has caused you to write again. I will go a little further now and say that I have the distinct impression that you are expecting more of an inquest than an inquest can deliver.

There are strict parameters laid down in law as to what can be investigated. The only four questions that an inquest can look at are the identity of the deceased and when, where and how he or she died. There are specific regulations designed to prevent an inquest becoming a substitute negligence claim, or a substitute complaint about care. There are avenues available for both of these and you appear to have explored one or other already.

My hope was that as Smith had recently been involved in an inquest that seemed to raise similar concerns as to those raised by Joshua's death, he might be able to at least have a conversation with the Newcastle Coroner about the case and prompt him to reconsider his decision. It was clear from this response that Mr Smith was not going to help us.

Given that the Newcastle Coroner had already set out his position, there seemed to be little point in pursuing this avenue any further. Instead, all my hopes for an independent investigation now rested with the Ombudsman.

In the meantime things were getting even more complicated. On August 7th Halsall forwarded me a letter he had written to the LSA in relation to their report into Joshua's care. The letter was supportive of our concerns and was extremely critical of the LSA. His concerns lay around four key points which I can summarise as follows:

- It was the Trust's Clinical Risk Manager who carried out the review on behalf of the LSA. How could she have been objective?

- The midwives were not questioned properly and the report dismisses Hoa remembering a temperature being recorded below 36° on the basis that the midwife would have called a doctor if that was the case

- The LSA did not discuss the case with the family

- The Trust were not asked to comment on the report and the LSA refused a request from them to be represented at the meeting between the LSA and the Titcombe family

Halsall's letter concluded:

Fundamental to this case is the fact that the midwives who were responsible for the care of Joshua failed to recognise, for a number of reasons, that he was ill. There were issues that should have alerted them to a potential problem that were missed. A good example being the fact that the baby did not manage to maintain his temperature. On more than one occasion Joshua was warmed up. I would find it quite distressing to believe that experienced midwives would feel that taking action repeatedly indicates a baby whose temperature is normal or that the room temperature was the cause of this fluctuation. The LSA report reports rather than challenges these events and uses them to vindicate the midwives of any accountability. I should however make it clear, that I do not disagree with the implications for practice and supervision for the midwives.

The letter left me with a genuine sense that Halsall was trying to do the right thing. It was strongly worded and it seemed clear that he was truly angry with the LSA for the way they had managed the report.

However, I was still confused by Halsall's overall response to us. Through my conversations with the Customer Services Manager I had recently learned that, during the Trust's investigation, the external 'experts' hadn't even interviewed the staff involved. The investigation had been carried out entirely on the basis of the statements which Halsall had been so reluctant to share with us. If Halsall had wanted the Trust's investigation to establish the full truth and to learn all possible lessons, why was the investigation he commissioned so superficial? Surely, an important part of any investigation process must be to formally interview the staff involved, if for no other reason than to understand their perspective about what happened and give them an opportunity to share any of their concerns. Was he holding something back?

I sent copies of this recent letter from Halsall to other organisations including the Ombudsman. Given that there was now clear disagreement about the sequence of events and the underlying causal factors leading to Joshua's death, I felt that the reasons for the Ombudsman to investigate were now overwhelming. We still had so many unanswered questions. We now knew that Joshua's death wasn't an isolated incident and that at least one other preventable death had happened shortly before.

Things started to move very quickly. The Nursing and Midwifery Council (NMC) had written to inform me that they would be carrying out their own investigation in relation to the fitness to practise of the midwives involved in Joshua's care. The LSA had confirmed that they were reviewing my complaint about the LSA report. I knew that the Ombudsman was nearing making a decision on whether to investigate. On top of all this Hoa's due date was getting closer and closer.

On August 13th, 2009 something odd happened. Out of the blue I received a call from the Trust's Medical Director. He sounded nervous but proceeded to explain that he was calling me because there had been a Data Protection Act (DPA) incident involving information relating to my wife and son that the Trust had a duty to inform me about. He went on to explain that a midwife who was being investigated by the Nursing and Midwifery Council had written a report about Joshua's care for the purposes of their investigation and that this report had been accidentally sent to an unknown external email address. In the context of everything else that we were facing at the time, we didn't think that a breach of DPA was a particularly serious matter. However, the Medical Director explained that it had been treated as a Serious Untoward Incident (SUI) and was being investigated.

A couple of days later I received a letter explaining the circumstances. It stated that the email correspondence was a 'purely professional' response to questions the NMC had asked about Joshua's case and 'nothing more'. I thought it was odd that a Trust that didn't declare Joshua's death as a 'SUI' until more than a month after he died would treat what seemed like a minor issue so seriously. Like so many other things I had been told by the Trust, I was to eventually learn that the truth was far more upsetting than I had been told.

The rest of August passed quickly. Originally the Ombudsman was going to make a decision on Joshua's case on August 12th, but I was told that the panel were still considering the case and it would be a matter of 'weeks not days' before I would find out. With this news I did my best to put all the issues on hold. Hoa was now nearing the end of her pregnancy and that was what I needed to concentrate on.

We made arrangements for Hoa's sister and her daughter, who live in Australia, to visit us in time for the birth. The whole family wanted Jessica's birth to be a time for healing and an opportunity to move forward. We did our best to be positive but this was a very anxious time for all. Before Joshua's death I am sure that we both would have anticipated the outcome of a healthy baby without a second thought, but now we were both scared. What if something happened during Jessica's birth? This would be too much for any of us to cope with. As a father, I wasn't going to take anything for granted this time. I would only accept the reality of our new baby when she was healthy and in my arms. As the due date approached this anxiety only increased.

On the September 22nd Hoa went into labour. There was a plan in place at Furness General and we had been given considerable reassurance regarding what would happen. The plan should ensure that no midwives involved in Joshua's care were involved in Jessica's birth but surely there was a chance of meeting some? I had so much sadness and anger at the dishonesty I'd been confronted with over the last year.

Before going to the hospital I made a firm personal resolution to place all of these issues on hold until Jessica was safely at home. The next few days had to be about Jessica and Hoa and nothing else.

When we arrived at the Maternity Unit, Hoa was examined in the same room she had been 11 months before. Jessica was born in the same room as Joshua. As planned, a doctor was present.

During the birth there was a moment when the umbilical cord was caught around Jessica's neck and had to be freed. It was a tense birth. After Jessica's head emerged there was what seemed liked a long delay before she was fully born. During this time, she suffered from what the midwife called 'compression' - she got a bit squashed and bruised. After Jessica was delivered she was transferred as planned straight to the Special Care Baby Unit. I watched as she was given precautionary antibiotics. A small injection with a syringe; it took only a few moments. I could not help but reflect on how straightforward this was. I felt a deep sadness that Joshua had been denied such a simple procedure.

Jessica and Hoa stayed at the Unit overnight and the care they both received was outstanding. The staff we met were kind and obviously aware of our situation.

The next day, September 23rd, 2009, I set out to FGH exactly as I had done on October 28th, 2008.

Only this time I got to take my wife and healthy baby home.

Chapter 6 - Lack of trust

Jessica brought us all a huge sense of joy. Hoa's sister and her daughter had arrived from Australia and stayed with us in our house. For the first time in months I saw happiness in Hoa and my mum and dad. I wrote a very appreciative letter to the Trust to thank the staff involved in Jessica's birth.

At the same time, the joy I felt with Jessica was tinged with a deep sense of sadness and guilt. While Jessica was warm and in the loving arms of her parents I couldn't help but reflect on how different things had been for Joshua and how easily his life could have been saved.

Jessica was not a substitute or replacement; our love and happiness for her were not a reason to give up on the answers I knew I still needed.

I now seemed to be wading through a quagmire of investigations into Joshua's death, none of them satisfactory.

Firstly there was Morecambe Bay Trust's own report, which was superficial to say the least and failed to acknowledge any discrepancies between the midwives' statements and what we had witnessed.

Secondly, the LSA report, examining failures of care by the midwives, written by the Trust's Risk Manager which turned out to be a whitewash (and criticised by the Trust's Chief Executive, Tony Halsall, himself).

Thirdly, the Maternity Unit who were bringing in their own external consultant. We hadn't heard from this yet.

Fourthly, Cumbria Police had started an investigation.

Fifthly, the CQC were assessing the hospital but couldn't deal with individual cases.

And sixthly – The Ombudsman, who still hadn't decided whether Joshua's case was going to be investigated or not.

In addition there was the Newcastle Coroner who had so far turned down our request for an inquest.

And there would be more to follow.

On October 29th, 2009 I finally received a response from the Ombudsman. The letter from Ann Abraham stated that she had spent some time discussing my complaints with the Care Quality Commission (CQC) and with Monitor and that:

In view of the oversight which the CQC are giving to the planned action of the Trust and the current position of Monitor, I am minded to decline to investigate your complaint. This is because I am satisfied that the CQC is the appropriate body to take action to ensure that the Trust carries out its plans to improve its service.

It went on to say that she had asked her Deputy, Kathryn Hudson, to visit me to explain the reasons behind her proposed decision and to give me an opportunity to express my views before she made her final decision.

I read the letter with a real sense of shock. I was certain, given the recent developments and the clarity with which I felt I had set out the serious unresolved issues, that the decision could only have been to investigate.

I first formally asked the Ombudsman to investigate on April 4th, 2009. It had taken Ann Abraham more than five months to suggest that she was 'not minded' to investigate.

I was also intrigued to know what Abraham was referring to in relation to the CQC and Monitor.

On November 1st I replied, accepting the offer to meet with Kathryn Hudson. My letter concluded:

We are very troubled that some of our most serious concerns about what happened to Joshua have still not been answered. We find it hard to understand how these aspects can be left unresolved without any further explanation or justification. I am sure the proposed meeting will help us to understand the reasons for your proposed decision and will also provide an opportunity for us to explain any outstanding concerns we might have.

Over the next few days I liaised with the Ombudsman's office and a date was agreed for the deputy Ombudsman, Kathryn Hudson, to visit us on Thursday 19th November.

When the day arrived my dad joined us at our home. I picked Kathryn up from the station and gave her a lift to our house.

Kathryn began by explaining that, through the Ombudsman's assessment of Joshua's case, she had spoken to the Care Quality Commission. They were aware that Morecambe Bay Trust was an organisation with serious problems, where functional and managerial weaknesses had let patients down. Kathryn said that these issues were not just limited to maternity services, but other areas too. These concerns had led to the CQC changing the Trust's rating from 'good' to 'fair' and that the CQC would not register the Trust until it was satisfied that standards had improved. Monitor, the organisation responsible for granting Foundation Trust status, would not do so until CQC had provided assurances that things had improved. This, we were told, would be a powerful mechanism to ensure improvements were made and lessons learned from Joshua's death.

This was a worrying statement. CQC was the regulator but I knew it did not have the power to investigate individual complaints. Why should the possible future actions of the CQC be any business of the Ombudsman in relation to their response to a complaint?

Kathryn went on to tell us that the Ombudsman was 'pleased' with the response Halsall had shown in relation to Joshua's death and that the Trust's action plan was 'robust and wide ranging'. We were told that the Trust was willing to share this action plan with us. Why had the Trust not already done this? The Ombudsman's confidence in Tony Halsall and the Trust's plan was clearly a key part of their decision, but how could anyone know that the Trust's action plan was sufficient or complete given that it was clear that a proper investigation had not taken place?

Kathryn brought with her a letter which set out the Ombudsman's thinking in more detail. The letter placed great emphasis on the role of the CQC and she was satisfied

'that the Trust have taken your concerns seriously and that CQC are taking action to monitor the situation at the Trust to ensure improvements are made'.

The letter went on:

I must stress that the work in maternity services at the Trust is being monitored by CQC and CQC will consider the Trust's application for registration with them very carefully to ensure standards are appropriate. In the meantime, the Trust will be unable to satisfy Monitor, the Foundation Trust Regulator, that they should achieve Foundation Trust status until they can demonstrate there has been sustained improvement.

In relation to the unresolved issues in Joshua's case, the letter stated:

It is clear to me that an investigation by my Office would not be able to give you the definitive answers you seek. As you know, Joshua's medical records are missing for the crucial first 24 hours of his life and while we could take action to interview the personnel involved in Joshua's care it is highly unlikely that we would be able to reach a firm finding on what took place and why.

It seemed incredible to me that Abraham was actually using that the fact that Joshua's critical medical records had gone missing as a reason not to investigate. Surely the opposite should have been the case?

The letter concluded:

I fully appreciate the importance of this matter to you and recognise that you will be disappointed that I am minded not to investigate your complaint. However, I hope that you will accept my reasons for that and that you will be reassured that your complaint has been taken extremely seriously by the Trust, CQC and Monitor and that efforts are already being made to improve the quality of service at the Trust.

Up until this point I was not aware of the extent to which CQC and Monitor were considering the circumstances of Joshua's death, so this news was welcome and reassuring.

However, where did this leave the many questions and concerns we still had? The Ombudsman appeared to have formed a view that the outstanding issues couldn't be resolved.

How was it possible to say this given that in reality, no proper investigation into the circumstances of Joshua's death had ever taken place?

The unresolved issues were many:

Why had the Trust's investigation not involved actually interviewing the staff involved in Joshua's care?

Why were the statements in relation to Joshua's death not taken until a month after his death?

Why were we only informed about the 'missing' observation chart several weeks later?

Why were we told that our chronology corresponded to the version of events reported by the midwives, when in fact there were huge discrepancies?

How would these discrepancies be resolved? They related to the preventable death of a child, surely they needed to be addressed?

What would be done about the LSA report which contained errors of fact relating to Joshua's death?

If all these issues were now abandoned, what message would this send to the NHS as a whole - that losing critical medical records and being dishonest about events that led to the preventable death of a child was acceptable?

We discussed all these issues with Kathryn but, as the meeting went on, it was clear that the Ombudsman's decision was not going to change. At the end of the meeting I made a desperate plea for Kathryn to take a strong message back to Ann Abraham to reconsider.

A few days later I sent a detailed letter to the Ombudsman setting out our concerns.

My letter concluded:

I can't do any more now than to ask you to consider the areas of concern I have detailed in this letter and urge you to help us move forward with these issues. I know that I cannot give up my fight for Joshua whilst denial and misinformation about his death prevails. I dearly hope that you won't either.

This hope was, of course, in vain.

Over the next few weeks I sent several more emails to Kathryn Hudson. I'm not ashamed to say they became increasingly desperate. I was literally begging her not to allow the Ombudsman to abandon Joshua's case. All other doors had led nowhere.

The Ombudsman now seemed the only hope we had of finding out what really happened to my son at Furness General. As was now routine, I updated all the other organisations I was in touch with, including the CQC, about the Ombudsman's preliminary decision.

On December 16th I received what was to be an important letter from the CQC's Regional Director. The letter began by acknowledging the care given to Joshua was 'highly unsatisfactory' and went on to state that although the CQC did not have the powers to investigate individual complaints, their remit was to question 'systemic failures in the operation of a Trust'. The letter outlined a number of particular concerns about UHMBT:

- The poor levels of multi-disciplinary work within maternity services at Barrow Hospital – particularly in respect of midwifery, obstetrics and paediatrics

- Poor evidence of effective communication and consistent working between maternity units located in the different UHMBT site

- Inadequate recording of the care provided to patients.

The CQC had warned the Chief Executive and Chair of the Trust that it needed to be able to demonstrate that it had made significant improvements in these areas before they would revise their internal risk rating of the Trust - Monitor take this rating into account when considering whether or not to award Foundation status to a Trust.

The letter went on to say that their powers to deal with Trusts was effectively limited to 'naming and shaming' but from April 1st, 2010 'the situation changes radically'. From that date all providers must register with the Commission, which in effect has to grant them 'licence to operate' – in extreme cases, they could make a Trust's continued operation illegal.

I had several thoughts about this letter.

Firstly, I was very alarmed that the CQC clearly had such serious concerns about the Maternity Unit at FGH. The letter warned 'We believe that if future tragedies are to be avoided, the Trust needs to be able to evidence a much more integrated approach to care'.

How could this be the case more than a year after Joshua's death?

The letter also referred to the tragic death of a baby in Milton Keynes that had been in the news recently, stating 'I imagine that this will resonate with your experience and cause you further distress'. Earlier in the month, the death of baby Ebony McCall at Milton Keynes maternity ward had been reported in the national news.

The report had followed an inquest into baby Ebony's death where the Coroner had been extremely critical of the Trust regarding staffing levels and the standard of care. The inquest came after an earlier Healthcare Commission investigation (the organisation that preceded the CQC) found a shortage of beds and midwives which meant some mothers were being discharged prematurely. The CQC had been quoted in the national media as being critical of the Trust's lack of progress.

The case had indeed caused me some distress. It was clearly absolutely right that baby Ebony's death was the subject of an inquest, but why had an inquest been refused into Joshua's death and why had there been no equivalent investigation at Furness General Hospital? What criteria did Coroners apply when deciding whether or not to open an inquest, and has this been applied consistently in Joshua's case?

After reading this, rather than feeling that the oversight of the CQC was a good reason for the Ombudsman to refuse to investigate, I felt even more strongly that it was an incontrovertible argument to do so.

Despite several more letters and phone calls I retained the strong sense that I was getting nowhere. It really did feel like the decision had been made and that nothing I said or did would change it.

Christmas came and went. It was now more than two months since I had been promised a final decision from the Ombudsman and more than a month since our meeting with Kathryn Hudson.

As my sense of injustice continued to grow I decided to try a new strategy. I prepared a document entitled 'Safety of Maternity Services at FGH'. The document put all the information I had at the time together. It made reference to the other baby deaths I knew about and the clear links with Joshua's case and also included details of CQC's recent letter to me. This included the current concerns about maternity services at Furness General and the information I now knew in relation to Monitor and Foundation status authorisation. The document concluded with a plea for an urgent investigation into the situation at the Trust.

I sent this together with the recent CQC letter to every organisation I was in touch with. I also sent a copy to the local paper who got back to me very quickly. Their reporter had made enquiries with the CQC and Monitor who had verified the situation. Furthermore, Monitor had confirmed that the decision to authorise the Trust for Foundation Trust status had been postponed.

The piece ran as a front page lead on January 15th, 2010. The headline was 'Lack of Trust'.

A health watchdog refused the trust which runs Furness General Hospital foundation trust status following a damning assessment of its midwifery services.

The University of Morecambe Bay Hospitals NHS Trust's application to become a foundation trust, which health bosses hoped would be approved this year, has been postponed by regulatory body Monitor.

This comes after investigations conducted following the death of newborn baby Joshua Titcombe over a year ago....

It went on to outline the story of Joshua's death and my complaint to the CQC. It reported how CQC had given a risk rating of the Trust's services as 'red' (then upgraded to 'amber'), how it assessed the poor levels of multi-disciplinary work within the maternity services and that the care provided to patients in maternity services was 'inadequate'. The Health Service Ombudsman would not comment due to confidentiality issues. It included these statements from Tony Halsall:

Around 1,200 babies are delivered safe and well at Furness General Hospital every year. Latest statistics show that Furness General Hospital and the trust as a whole are among the safest places in England to have a baby...

After baby Joshua died, I said we would ensure that a full, externally managed, investigation would be carried out into maternity services at Furness General Hospital. This was to see what could be improved and ensure we took steps to make those improvements...

Today, Furness General Hospital is a safer place to have a baby as a result of the lessons learned from the external investigation.

I was pleased with the piece and knew that it would have a big impact. I was also deeply angry about the Trust's press statement. Halsall had said, 'Every member of staff has taken this as a learning experience and been totally open, honest and fully co-operative with the investigation'. This could not have been further from the truth.

In reality, Joshua's critical medical records had gone missing and, in the absence of contemporary records, staff had reported events that my wife and I knew for certain were not true.

Halsall had stated: 'Latest statistics show that Furness General Hospital and the Trust as a whole are among the safest places in England to have a baby'.

Evidence was mounting that this simply couldn't be the case. I would later learn that the statistics Halsall was referring to excluded deaths such as Joshua's - although Joshua was clearly failed by FGH, he died outside the Trust.

It would eventually be shown just how wrong Halsall was. At the time this press statement was issued, 'significant risks' to the lives of mothers and babies were continuing.

In the following years more lives were to be lost.

Chapter 7 - Closing doors

Just a few days after the press report yet more significant and troubling information came to light. My father had received a phone call from a Carl Hendrickson (unlike us, my mum and dad were in the phone book). Carl told him how in 2008, just a few months before Joshua's death, his wife and baby son had died following childbirth at FGH. Carl had read the report about Joshua's death in the local paper and felt compelled to make contact – it was far too similar to his own experiences.

A few days later I had a long phone conversation with Carl. He described tragic and deeply traumatic events. His wife had suffered a 'fit' during childbirth and had collapsed and died as a consequence of a complication known as 'Amniotic Fluid Embolism'. Carl's son, Chester, had been delivered by emergency Caesarean section. Although Carl had originally been reassured by a doctor that his baby was fine, baby Chester was subsequently transferred in a critical condition to another hospital where he died. As in Joshua's case, this was another baby death that was excluded from the Trust's neonatal mortality figures.

These events were clearly horrific but it would not be until many years later that Carl would eventually establish the truth in relation to the avoidable failures that occurred.

Carl described some things that caused immediate alarm.

He described how, when his wife appeared to have a 'fit', he had asked for the midwife to call a doctor. The response was, 'We don't need no doctors here'.

This seemed to me to be yet more evidence of what the Coroner had described as 'the midwives running the show'.

More worrying still, following the tragic loss of his wife and son, medical records had gone missing including a critical Cardiac Trace recording.

This was to be the start of a long friendship with Carl whose help, support and encouragement throughout the years since have been invaluable.

Following this conversation with Carl, the first thing I did was make sure that the Ombudsman was aware of this new information. However, any hope that this would make a difference was short lived.

On February 3rd, 2010 I received the letter from Ann Abraham I feared. The letter confirmed the provisional decision that the Ombudsman would not investigate Joshua's death.

The explanation was as follows:

First, with regard to your concerns about the general quality of care at the Trust, it is clear that the organisation, and in particular Tony Halsall, the Chief Executive, have taken those concerns very seriously and have acknowledged that the level of care given to Joshua fell far below acceptable standards. You told one of my Assessors, Harriet Clover, that you wanted to ensure that the risks to other mothers and babies were reduced. The Trust has commissioned two investigations and I have asked one of my clinical advisers to look at the midwifery strategy put in place as a result. She tells me that the strategy is comprehensive and robust and is supported by an appropriate action plan which covers the recommendations of the external review and the Local Supervising Authority (LSA) report.

Phrases like 'the strategy is comprehensive and robust and is supported by an appropriate action plan' rang hollow in my ears. Is this really going to stop more babies dying? Did it mean anything at all?

On the role of the CQC and Monitor:

One of our concerns has been to make sure that the CQC was fully aware of the issues arising from Joshua's death and was actively overseeing the work of the Trust on its action plan. The CQC does indeed have the Trust closely under review and is looking to see positive outcomes from the action plan before its concerns will be reduced...

The Trust is currently unable to satisfy Monitor, the Foundation Trust Regulator, that it should achieve Foundation Trust status, and this provides another impetus for the Trust to implement the action plan effectively. In summary, I am satisfied that the action plan, together with the close oversight of the CQC, will ensure that lessons have been learnt and improvements made and that an investigation by my Office is unlikely to achieve any more in this area.

The letter went on to discuss the discrepancies in the mid-wives' accounts:

As you know, despite thorough searches, the records for the first 24 hours of Joshua's life are still missing. The staff involved have been interviewed on more that one occasion. It is unlikely that they would now change their accounts of the events and for this reason, in the absence of records, a further investigation is not likely to reach a firm finding of what took place and why.

This was the death of a child. How could the fact that critical records were missing and that staff were unlikely to 'change their accounts of the events' possibly be an acceptable reason not to investigate?

The letter notes that I had a complaint outstanding with the LSA in relation to their report and stated:

If the LSA is unable to resolve your complaint you can of course return to me in relation to this aspect of your concerns at that time.

The final paragraph of the letter read:

In conclusion, the improvements currently being put in place by the Trust and monitored by CQC are extensive and are a testament to the efforts you have put into ensuring that Joshua's death has achieved a positive outcome in preventing others from suffering as you and your family have done. While I do not think that an investigation could add significantly to what you have already achieved, I hope that you will be able to accept my reasons and take reassurance from this letter that your concerns have not been dismissed lightly by anyone in this organisation and least of all by myself.

Although I knew what was coming, when I read the letter I could do nothing for a while but sit and cry. When something as awful as Joshua's death had happened, followed by so much dishonesty and so many unanswered questions, how could the Ombudsman, the only organisation in the entire hierarchy of the NHS with the power to properly investigate, refuse to do so?

A few days later I replied:

For reasons I will try and outline in this letter, I find your decision deeply unsatisfactory and untenable.

You state that 'despite thorough searches, the records for the first 24 hours of Joshua's life are still missing. The staff have been interviewed on more than one occasion. It is unlikely that they would now change their accounts of the events and for this reason, in the absence of records, a further investigation is not likely to reach a firm finding of what took place and why.'

I am flabbergasted that this can be given as a reason not to investigate. Surely these facts are overwhelming reasons to investigate? These events relate to the preventable death of a child. Are you really suggesting that it is acceptable to leave the events that led to Joshua's death open ended, simply because the records have gone missing and the staff are sticking to their story?

You say that the 'staff have been interviewed on more than one occasion'. I have a conversation on record, with [The Trust's Customer Care Manager], whereby she told me that during the 'external' investigation, not a single member of staff was interviewed. The only interviews I am aware of were undertaken by the LSA, whose involvement in this case, even the Trust has criticised for lacking objectivity...

...You are certain that these discrepancies cannot be resolved, yet you are also aware that no proper process has ever been undertaken to try... To pre-empt that any investigation 'is not likely to reach a firm finding of what took place and why', is not an acceptable reason for you to refuse to try.

...In closing the door on us, this is now the final word on Joshua's life. No criticisms, no recommendations and no chance for us to ever get the answers we need.

...My son was taken away from me, but the saddest memory is not his death, but the events that took place afterwards.

I have begged and begged for your help, not because I want compensation, not because I think you can bring Joshua back, but because I genuinely don't want to see any other family go through the experience we have. I believe with all my heart that you have missed an opportunity to ensure that what happened after Joshua died, is never repeated again. If the Trust has nothing to hide, they would have welcomed an inquiry with open arms. The least it would have achieved is comfort and reassurance to my family and the wider community that a process has been followed...

Medical records have gone missing, lies have been told. If this can go on unchallenged, then I don't think there is any hope for the NHS in the future.

Please re-think your decision.

My efforts to appeal the Ombudsman's decision not to investigate would prove to be futile, but the battle to ensure the truth about what happened to my son and the scale of problems at FGH was far from over.

Chapter 8 - Hope at last

The decision of the Ombudsman not to investigate had left me with a growing sense of anger and injustice. These issues had now completely taken over every aspect of my life.

Even at this stage my feelings towards Halsall were mixed. I began to form the hypothesis that while I believed he had made genuine attempts to ensure there was learning from Joshua's death, he was compromised by the reality of being Chief Executive of the Trust and ultimately responsible for the progress of the organisation's 'strategic objectives'. The most important of these appeared to be achieving Foundation Trust status.

On February 5th, 2010, just days after receiving the letter confirming that the Ombudsman had refused to investigate, I decided that I would write again to Mitford, the Coroner in Newcastle. I had been thinking more about the Milton Keynes case and I felt that I had to explore the reasons why an inquest into Joshua's death had been refused.

On February 10th Mitford responded with a holding letter acknowledging receipt and confirming that he would be responding again once he had reviewed the previous documentation. A few days later I received a full response.

Having considered matters very carefully, I take the view that I cannot now open an inquest into the death of your son Joshua. At the time the death was reported to me and my officers made the appropriate investigations, it was clear that the cause of Joshua's death was a natural cause and where this is the situation then a Coroner does not have jurisdiction to proceed further towards an inquest.

The letter went on:

Although you have now raised a variety of concerns, none of them were made known to my officer at the time but, in any event, I do not feel they would have been matters which would have led to me opening an inquest. They are matters which would, if you wish to pursue them, be the subject of appropriate procedures to deal with this sort of situation.

A few days later on February 18th I wrote back, challenging Mitford's statement that the cause of Joshua's death was 'natural':

I do not see how the death of a baby, who from birth, never left the care of an NHS hospital, from an entirely preventable condition, can be seen as 'natural'. If someone is walking down a street and a brick falls on their head and they bleed to death on the pavement, the facts could quickly be established that the cause of the death was bleeding from the head – does this mean that you wouldn't hold an inquest to find out why the brick fell in the first place?

I attached some press releases, including the Milton Keynes case, in support of my argument that the circumstances of Joshua's death really ought to have triggered an inquest.

This was a busy time. The correspondence with the Newcastle Coroner was only one of the negotiations I was involved in.

The North West Strategic Health Authority (NWSHA) had been in contact with me in relation the complaint I had made about the LSA report. At the time, the NWSHA was the organisation responsible for the midwifery supervisory system and therefore they were addressing my complaint. On February 19th two managers from the NWSHA visited me at my home to discuss the case. They told me that the NWSHA had asked a senior midwife from another LSA to review the investigation report into Joshua's case. I was happy with this suggestion and hoped that this process might at least lead to the LSA report into Joshua's death being reconsidered.

On February 26th Mitford replied to my further letter. This time, Mitford's letter took a slightly different tone.

As I indicated to you in my last letter, I did not feel that there was any further evidence presented to me to contradict the original cause of death supplied and therefore I could not be satisfied that I had jurisdiction to open an inquest. Whilst I appreciate the concerns you have expressed, if I am to consider opening an inquest, even at this very late stage, there must be clear evidence on which I could make that decision.

…It is only if new evidence of facts which were not previously available to me and may suggest the need for an inquest that I would have jurisdiction to reconsider.

…I emphasise again that if I am to consider further the opening of an inquest, I need detailed factual evidence. The matters you have raised in your previous correspondence fall far short of the factual detail I would require.

The letter concluded by setting out that if I wished Mr Mitford to further consider opening an inquest I needed to supply such evidence as well as a '...detailed statement...

setting out your recollection of what happened to Joshua whilst he was cared for in the hours before his collapse'.

For the first time it appeared that there was at least a glimmer of hope, but I couldn't help reflect on how unfair the burden of proof seemed to be. Here I was, knowing that critical medical records relating to Joshua had gone missing, that the Ombudsman had refused to investigate and that the Trust's own investigation had not even involved interviewing the staff concerned, and yet the burden of responsibility was now on me to provide 'detailed factual evidence'. The very reason I wanted an inquest was because such detailed factual evidence relating to Joshua's death was proving almost impossible to obtain.

Over the next couple of weeks I worked on my response. I knew this would be a crucial letter and I wanted to set out the facts, evidence and arguments as clearly as I possibly could.

On March 6th I sent a four-page letter to Mitford's office. I enclosed copies of the Trust's investigation, the original chronology of events my wife and I wrote shortly after Joshua's death, the LSA report and the PowerPoint presentation I had prepared.

My letter explained what had been accepted and on what evidence, the conflicts in the accounts and my key outstanding concerns. I gave the letter all I had. This really did seem like the last possible chance of finding out the full truth about what had happened to my son.

In the following weeks contact with Halsall continued. I asked for the opportunity to discuss the Trust's internal report with the external experts who had written it.

Halsall was insistent that this would not happen. How could this be reasonable? Surely the authors of the report should be prepared to discuss their work and findings with the family?

On March 19th, 2010 Halsall sent me a letter which he described as 'drawing the complaints process to an end', accepting that the Trust had failed Joshua and that this had led to my family receiving 'substantial compensation'. The letter went on:

You are aware of my personal involvement in Joshua's case and of how seriously I have taken your concerns throughout. However, having exhausted the complaints process, including review by the Ombudsman and having had an apology and financial compensation, I must now draw the complaints process to an end. Nothing I can say or do and no level of financial compensation can ever bring Joshua back and for that I will always be extremely sorry.

I have commented previously about how much has happened since Joshua's death in terms of making services safer not only at FGH but across all of our maternity units for which you should be proud that you have represented Joshua so vigorously.

The letter concluded:

We will continue to work with the reviewing agencies to achieve their outcomes and I will update you on the further progress against the action plan... I will not, however, enter into further correspondence about the reports and conclusions already completed.

The letter stated that Halsall was willing to meet me to discuss further.

Again, like so much of my contact with Halsall in the past, I had mixed feelings about his letter. Halsall seemed sincere in his belief that improvements had been made following Joshua's death. But he was also aware of the significant discrepancies and unanswered questions and that a proper process of investigation had not been followed.

I was angered that he had referred to 'significant compensation'. We had accepted an offer of compensation from the NHSLA in 2009 but this really was inconsequential. I would gladly have given up all the money and possessions we owned to have Joshua back.

With the possibility of an Ombudsman's investigation now completely removed, Halsall was free to draw the complaints process to an end and to refuse to correspond with me any further regarding the Trust's investigations, reports and conclusions. It seemed that I had nowhere else to turn and that every door I had tried was now closed.

However, my sense of frustration and helplessness was soon to be relieved.

Just a few days later, on March 24th, I received a letter from the Newcastle Coroner that was to change everything.

The letter stated that Mitford had now had the opportunity to consider the full information which I had presented:

That information now leads me to the view that there is evidence which needs to be considered about the events, circumstances and treatment of Joshua at Furness General Hospital and that it is therefore appropriate for an inquest into his death to be opened.

I couldn't believe what I was reading. Finally, 19 months after I lost Joshua, I now knew that a respected process of investigation that could properly establish the truth was going to happen. With tears in my eyes, I read the rest of the letter.

I therefore propose to open an inquest as soon as possible and I propose, in view of the distance between Newcastle and your place of residence, that the opening process could be achieved administratively without the need for you to travel a considerable distance to attend the opening which would only deal with the formality of confirmation of identification -- a matter which has never been an issue in this situation.

If you therefore agree, I will open the inquest without your attendance and will then consult my colleague Mr Ian Smith, Coroner in South Cumbria on the issue of whether it may be appropriate for the inquest to be transferred to be dealt with in his jurisdiction.

I felt a huge sense of relief after reading this letter. In his last letter, Halsall had said that he was no longer prepared to '…enter into further correspondence about the reports and conclusions already completed'. Whether Halsall liked it or not, this news meant that the unresolved issues associated with Joshua's death would now have to be confronted.

Over the next few days the inquest was opened and, as suggested, Mitford liaised with my local Coroner, Ian Smith. During this period, anxious to know that things were progressing to plan, I phoned Smith's office a number of times and spoke to his assistant who was helpful and happy to keep me informed.

On April 1st I received a letter from Smith confirming that the jurisdiction had been transferred. However, the tone of the letter left me feeling hurt and upset.

It began with a brief paragraph stating that Smith had now accepted jurisdiction for Joshua's inquest. It then proceeded to set out a number of 'matters' he needed me to 'understand right from the outset'. These included:

The investigation is the Coroner's investigation not the family's investigation and I must make it clear that I will direct the course of the investigation in accordance with my legal obligations.

I assure you that we will carry out the investigation as quickly and as thoroughly as we can, but please do not telephone in the way that you have in the past. We are an investigation service; we are not a bereavement or counselling service.

The inquest is designed to investigate the primary facts. It is not an investigation into the appropriateness or thoroughness of other investigations that may have taken place, nor is it a mechanism for this and if you wish to do so you should make a complaint if you have not already done so. That is quite separate from an inquest.

For better or for worse the system is that the Coroner investigates individual death. It may be argued that this is a fault with the system but none-the-less it is the Law and it is not possible or appropriate to start linking one death with another death in anything other than an indirect fashion.

The purpose of the Inquest, as defined by statute (Section 11(5) Coroners Act, 1988, and rule 36 Coroners Rules, 1984) is to establish the answer to four questions namely, who was the deceased and how, when and where did that person come by his death. The inquest cannot go beyond that remit.

The letter concluded:

I do not anticipate that the Health Authority will respond to me inside at least two weeks, and probably longer. When I do hear from them I will have a considerable amount of work to do to see where the investigation is going to go from that basis and I will keep you informed of progress, via my Coroner's Officer, as and when I can but this will not be daily.

I could only conclude that Smith had formed a view that I was a difficult or unreasonable person and that I needed to be put in my place at an early stage. At this time, I had never met Smith or his assistant. To this day I don't fully understand why this initial contact was so negative. I drafted a very angry letter in response but, after reflecting on what this would achieve, decided not to send it. Smith was now the only hope we had. What he thought and how he treated me was irrelevant as long as he carried out a thorough investigation.

The stress of constantly thinking about Joshua and fighting battles was taking its toll. My relationship with Hoa was becoming strained. We had a young baby in the house and much of my energy was being spent fighting Joshua's case. I was also holding down a responsible job managing several complex and high value contracts for a large nuclear project. This now involved regular trips to the US to visit suppliers. I no longer had a social life and I was losing interest in everything outside the case. It was around this time, following advice from family and my GP, that I decided to seek some professional help.

I had private medical insurance as part of my employment contract and I arranged to see a local counsellor on a private basis. During these sessions I was assessed for Post Traumatic Stress Disorder and the scores not only confirmed I was suffering from this but put me towards the extreme end of the scale. I subsequently had regular sessions using Cognitive Behavioural Therapy.

Throughout this time I also continued correspondence with the Trust. Halsall's last letter included an offer to meet; given that, since I'd last met Halsall, an inquest had been opened and the situation had moved forward, I decided to take up the offer. A meeting was arranged at Westmorland General Hospital in Kendal.

The meeting went ahead on May 21st. My father accompanied me. I had made a decision to record the meeting on my mobile phone. This proved to be important. The meeting covered a wide range of issues. I discussed how the Trust would prepare for the inquest and whether the Trust would have legal representation and a barrister. Halsall told me that they would, but that the involvement of the legal team would be minimal. It seemed very unfair that the Trust would have access to funds to provide professional representation but Joshua's family did not.

I also discussed with Halsall my concerns about the other cases I knew about and their clear similarities to Joshua's case. Halsall responded by saying that the Trust did not accept responsibility for any of the other cases and argued strongly that they were unavoidable events in which the staff at the Unit managed well.

Halsall also spoke in some detail about the changes that had been made at the Maternity Unit at Furness General and his confidence that the Unit was now much safer as a consequence of the actions taken following Joshua's death. He told me that the CQC had closely scrutinised the service and stated that there was 'nothing the CQC don't know about our organisation, or that we have not shared with them completely and openly'. These words came out smoothly, as if it was a rehearsed line.

It was later to emerge that this was far from the truth, and in circumstances that would leave the CQC, Monitor and the general public shocked.

Chapter 9 - 'NMC Shit'

In May 2010 there had been a General Election which unseated the Labour government. We now had a Con-Lib Dem Coalition government. By this time, my local MP John Hutton had made a decision to retire from politics and we had a new MP, John Woodcock.

On June 4th I made contact with John Woodcock's office. I provided as much information as I could and I asked if we could arrange to meet.

I was very aware that during the inquest we would not have any legal representation unless we funded it ourselves. Why was this something tax payers' money would provide for the Trust and yet no representation was available for families like ours? This really did seem like a huge unfairness and an imbalance in the system.

Over the next few weeks I looked into the possibility of paying for legal representation myself. I made contact with the solicitors who Carl told me were helping to progress his ongoing legal case. The solicitors were supportive and helpful from my first contact.

I was also told that there was a system administered through the Ministry of Justice which offered 'exceptional funding' to cover representation at inquests. However, this was only applied to cases which satisfied something called 'Article 2' of the Human Rights Act and was only granted on very rare occasions. For example, the families of the victims of Harold Shipman were not granted exceptional funding for their inquests. I was desperate and running out of options so I agreed to pay the fees necessary for my solicitor to submit the application.

Low times came and went but the week starting June 7th was a particularly tough one. Things between Hoa and I were difficult. I had become increasingly frustrated at the situation and the stress was becoming too much. I had become so focused on my battle with the hospital that I had little time for anything else. It must have felt to Hoa like she had lost her husband as well as her son. I had a long chat with my mum and dad and they gave me strong advice to take a step back and let the inquest take its course.

On June 10th I was so stressed that I took the day off work. I sent an email to the Customer Care Manager explaining that I wanted to take a step back and look after the family that I still had.

Years later I obtained some internal documents from the Trust relating to how they responded to this email. The content was deeply hurtful.

In fact I didn't take a step back but I carried on pushing for answers. I'm very glad that I did.

On June 18th I heard from the Nursing and Midwifery Council. It was now 19 months after Joshua's death and some 16 months since I had first written to the NMC about Joshua's case. The email read:

...I have spoken to my manager and he confirms that our investigation/process is on hold pending the results on the inquest.

The NMC stated on its website that its job was to 'protect the health and wellbeing of the public'. How effective the NMC could possibly be in this function, if its investigatory procedures, following failures in care as serious as those in Joshua's case, took so long to progress? It would be several months before the inquest was held - surely the NMC ought to progress its investigations sooner than this?

On June 25th I received a letter from Mike Farrar, the Chief Executive of the North West Strategic Health Authority, along with a copy of the review of the LSA report into Joshua's death.

The review concluded:

On completion of a thorough review of the LSA supervisory report and the actions taken by the SoMs [Supervisors of Midwives] responsible for formulating the report - as well as interviewing the author – I am in no doubt that the actions taken were in line with the LSA policy in use at the time and indeed are consistent with the National Guidelines developed by the LSAMO UK Forum adopted for national use by all LSAs within the United Kingdom in January 2009.

I believe that the recommendations made by the SoMs responsible for investigating each individual midwife's practice, are consistent with good statutory supervision. I believe it is commendable that a SoM investigation was initiated as soon as a serious untoward incident was known and that midwifery practice issues identified as requiring further investigation.

In my opinion, it is also commendable, that from this supervisory investigation sixteen recommendations were made with regard to midwifery practice and service provider roles and responsibilities. I am of the opinion that the recommendations made by the investigating SoMs regarding individual midwives' practice are consistent with evidence gathered throughout the investigation and reflective of the SoMs competence in fulfilling the roles and responsibilities of a SoM which are around protecting the public by empowering midwives and midwifery students to practise safely and effectively.

My complaint about the LSA report into Joshua's death included that the author had discounted the version of events that my wife and I had recalled (for example, the temperatures my wife had seen on Joshua's observation chart, Joshua's condition at birth and the fact that we knew an overhead heater had been used directly above Joshua). The report evaded these issues altogether.

In my opinion from the evidence available it was clear that all correspondence received by the Local Supervising Authority Midwifery Officer (LSAMO) Marian Drazek, from Mr Titcombe – in which questions were raised – was subsequently passed to the investigating SoMs, in order that all necessary information could be gathered, to allow an evidence based response to be made from the Local Supervising Authority (LSA).

The letter from Mike Farrar of the NWSHA seemed to be satisfied by this:

You will see from her report that our reviewer does confirm that the Local Supervising Authority function had followed proper process in conducting the original investigation on the actions of midwives. The reviewer has commended the fact that following the investigation a total of 16 recommendations had been made with regard to midwifery practice and service provider roles and responsibilities and these have been implemented. It has been confirmed that the actions taken were in line with the Local Supervising Authority policy and national guidelines in place at the time.

My initial reaction to reading this report and the letter from Farrar was outrage and anger. What I was reading was, again, a complete whitewash. It didn't address any of the issues which I had raised and, furthermore, it had even pretty much discounted the issues that Halsall himself, the Chief Executive of the Trust, had formally raised about the supervisory investigation into Joshua's death. On further reflection, I calmed down and thought things through rationally.

This report was so obviously lacking in objectivity that it simply wasn't credible. I was sure that anyone with even a basic understanding of the events who looked at it would instantly see that this was the case.

The events that followed were to prove that my instincts were right.

After receiving the report I constructed a letter that took apart, point by point, the logic and conclusion of the SHA's review.

I sent the letter to Farrar. I also copied my letter to the Head of Midwifery at the NMC, Christina McKenzie.

Whenever I look back on Joshua's story there are moments when it felt as if the entire system was closing ranks to keep the truth hidden. At moments like these I was lucky enough to gain support from some individuals who just at the right time provided the support and challenge needed to push back. Christina McKenzie was one such person.

Over the following few days I discussed Joshua's case with Christina. She was obviously appalled. In my telephone conversations with her she told me that the lack of objectivity in the review was obvious. The NMC were now involved. In the following weeks conversations took place between the NWSHA and the NMC which eventually resulted in a decision by the NMC that a second review into the LSA report was necessary. Farrar was later to confirm this by letter.

On August 2nd I received a response from my request for the Ombudsman to review their decision not to investigate Joshua's case. The review decision was well written and thoughtful but, perhaps inevitably, it supported the original decision that Ann Abraham had made. As we had now secured an inquest, it argued this was a further reason why an Ombudsman's investigation was not needed.

Over the next few weeks I spent a lot of time reflecting on the situation. The opening of an inquest was a huge relief, but this was tempered by the negative correspondence I'd had with the Coroner. While the Trust would have access to expensive expert legal representation we would only have the Coroner to rely on. The tone of his correspondence gave me little confidence. Joshua's critical medical records had gone missing and it was clear that the hospital staff in their statements had not told the full truth in relation to what happened. Furthermore, the NWSHA had just carried out a review of the LSA report which supported the process and the conclusions. Even though this had been challenged and a second review was being established, how was this going to affect the inquest?

The more I thought about these issues, the more I became incensed about the injustice of the situation. My grief for Joshua remained huge. This was affecting every aspect of my life. I'd lost my son. It wasn't right that my family and myself were still suffering because of these issues. I was becoming more and more distressed.

On August 18th I decided to do something to at least make people aware of these injustices. I prepared an A4 poster with the title 'Missing Medical Records Baby Joshua Titcombe'. The poster offered a reward of £1,000 and provided the contact number for Cumbria Police. These were actions that, with hindsight, I regret but at the time I was simply too desperate to care.

Late that evening I printed and laminated around a dozen copies of the poster and went to FGH. First I visited the management offices and put posters up on the doors and notice board. I then went to other areas of the hospital, including the Special Care Baby Unit, where I had been told that Joshua's records had last been seen. I left the hospital and drove home.

The next day I awoke to an email from the Trust's Customer Services Manager. It was a fairly polite message telling me that the posters had been removed and asking me not to take 'direct action' again. That evening I had a knock on the door and answered it to a police officer holding a photocopy of the poster. I was expecting a confrontation but, in fact, the officer could not have been nicer. The police had received a complaint from the Trust but his main concern was that I had used the number for Cumbria Police and advised me to use my own phone number in future. He told me that he and his colleagues in Barrow had huge sympathy for my situation.

I remained in contact with DCS Goulding, providing him with regular updates. I found an article on-line about a case involving a preventable death due to clinical failure that was subject to a full corporate manslaughter investigation. I wrote a detailed letter to Goulding setting out what I felt were the parallels with Joshua's case.

Although I did not know it at the time, the view of Cumbria Police was now starting to change.

Over the next few weeks I put a lot of thought into the issue of legal representation for the inquest. I had written to the Chief Executive of the NHS Litigation Authority, Steven Walker, who responded kindly, but set out his position that the NHSLA would not be able to help. However, Steven followed up to tell me about a scheme that the charity Action against Medical Accidents (AvMA) were running, which provided help to people in exactly the situation I was in. AvMA had already provided me with useful advice shortly after Joshua's death. Steven emailed the Chief Executive of AvMA, Peter Walsh, and I followed up with an email.

Peter was extremely helpful and offered to see if a barrister signed up with their scheme would be willing to provide representation at Joshua's inquest free of charge.

Following this development, I had further discussions with my solicitors. I had put in an application for exceptional funding but knew that the chances of getting this were extremely slim. I discussed the offer of help from AvMA and my solicitors also agreed to see if they could source a barrister from the contacts they had who was willing to provide representation on a pro bono (free) basis.

On August 24th I had some good news. My solicitor confirmed they had found a barrister who was willing to help. I mentioned, earlier in this book, the important moments in Joshua's story when specific individuals changed the course of events. This was another of those moments. The barrister was Paula Sparks; her professionalism, expertise and passion were to make a strong contribution to the effective presentation of information to the Coroner.

My solicitors agreed to provide the help we needed during the inquest on an expenses only basis, providing I paid the upfront legal costs associated with the inquest preparations. While this was still a significant sum of money, it meant we had an affordable way forward that I felt would provide the very best chance of securing the truth for Joshua. This was a huge weight off my mind.

A few weeks later important news also emerged about the Morecambe Bay Trust. On October 1st, 2010 it was announced that the Trust had achieved Foundation Trust status.

The article published by the Trust on its website stated:

University Hospitals of Morecambe Bay NHS Trust (UHMBT) has been awarded Foundation Trust (FT) status, effective from today.

Monitor, the independent body which regulates NHS FTs, approved the Trust's application at its Board meeting on Wednesday. UHMBT is only the third acute NHS Trust in the country to be awarded FT status by Monitor this year...

The application and approval process involved an extremely detailed assessment into the Trust's financial plans, quality of services and governance structure by a number of external organisations including Monitor, the Care Quality Commission, the Department of Health and PricewaterhouseCoopers...

It has been a long journey for the Trust - three years ago, it was £6.5m in debt and is now debt free. Over that time, the Trust's performance has also improved – this is highlighted by the green risk rating awarded from the Care Quality Commission and the Auditor's Local Evaluation score of four – which is equivalent to 'excellent'.

Tony Halsall, Chief Executive, UHMBT, said: 'This is a really important day for us. Achieving FT status not only acknowledges the significant progress we have made but gaining this external validation following such an in-depth and detailed assessment process is an indication of our clinical and financial stability'.

I had mixed feelings about the news. Seeing the Trust celebrating its achievements when we were still suffering so much as a consequence of its failures felt hurtful but, at the same time, this seemed like a clear indication that genuine improvements had been made. How else could CQC and Monitor have allowed the authorisation to go ahead?

In mid October 2010 we took a family holiday for four weeks to Vietnam. This was a chance to see Hoa's family and, I hoped, a time to switch off and relax for a while. The holiday was a lovely and welcome break. It brought back memories of when Hoa and I had met all those years ago. So much had changed in our lives since then.

The holiday passed quickly and, soon after I returned, I was invited to a meeting with the North West Strategic Health Authority to discuss the review of the original LSA report. On November 19th I travelled to the NWSHA's offices in Manchester to meet with the review team and Mike Farrar, the Chief Executive. Hoa and my dad came with me.

The first thing I noticed when I arrived at the offices was just how swish they were. It was a very modern building of stainless steel and glass construction. It was immaculate and luxurious and I couldn't help but think about how much it must have cost to build.

We were taken to a room and offered tea and coffee and then given a presentation of the review work that had been undertaken between the NWSHA and the NMC. It soon became clear that the NWSHA's position had now changed.

There was now an acknowledgment that the original supervisory investigation into Joshua's death had been significantly delayed. The investigation should have started straight away but it was put on hold for 5 months while the Trust's investigation progressed. This latest review had found that the boundaries of the remit of the LSA report had become 'blurred' and that, because the report was written by the Trust's Maternity Risk Manager, it was not independent. Most importantly, this latest review had concluded that the LSA report 'lacked logic' and that evidence was 'not clearly presented so as to support the conclusions'.

This was an immense relief. At last it seemed as if the tide of obstruction might be turning. Before we left we were told that Farrar would be formally writing to me to confirm the findings of the review and that, since the LSA report had been shared with the NMC and the Coroner, the NWSHA would be writing to both to share the conclusion that the LSA report was significantly flawed.

I received the letter from Mike Farrar a few weeks later. This confirmed what we had been told.

Now that the NWSHA had accepted that the LSA report into Joshua's death was flawed, I started to wonder what the next actions would be. A few weeks later I wrote back to Farrar and asked him that, if he now accepted that a proper supervisory investigation into Joshua's death had never taken place, would he now ensure that such a process would be undertaken as soon as possible. I was not to receive a response for some time.

In early December, while thinking about the inquest and all that I'd been through since Joshua's death, I remembered the phone call I had received in mid 2009 from the Medical Director of the Trust about a DPA issue. At the time I was told the incident involved a report written by one of the midwives for the NMC which had been accidentally sent to an erroneous email address. The Medical Director told me that the email and the report it contained by the midwife were 'purely professional' and that there was 'nothing more' to the incident.

However, as I also remembered being told that the incident was being handled under the Trust's Serious Untoward Incident (SUI) policy, I decided to make a formal request for a copy of the SUI report.

On January 7th, 2011 the Trust's Customer Services Manager emailed me a copy of this document. I opened it on my home PC (it was in MS-Word format) and began to read it. Large sections were redacted, but this redacted version appeared to support what I had been told by the Medical Director. It was a report written for the NMC about the circumstances of Joshua's death, which had been accidentally emailed to an incorrect email address (the email address used was just one character different to the intended email address).

However, as I clicked around with the mouse on the Word document all the redactions suddenly disappeared.

When I re-read it I could not believe what it revealed. The midwife had attached a report she had written about Joshua's care to an email she was forwarding under the title, 'NMC Shit'. This, about my beautiful baby boy who I had to watch die in the most horrific circumstances. His death had turned my world upside down. How could a midwife responsible for his care title an email containing a report relating to his death, 'NMC Shit'?

Furthermore, why had the Trust's Medical Director told me that this correspondence was 'comprehensive', 'professional' and 'nothing more'?

If it weren't for the fact that I had accidentally removed the redactions I would have been none the wiser about its true nature. Why would the Trust be covering up such an appalling incident?

That evening I phoned Carl to tell him about what had happened. I broke down in tears over the phone. It just seemed too awful to be true. How could anyone aware of Joshua's death behave in this way?

Following this I made a formal request to the Trust for copies of all documents, emails and reports that mentioned Joshua or any member of my family. I had learned that this was called a Subject Data Access Request (SDAR) - something anyone is entitled to ask any public body for under the Data Protection Act (DPA).

If this is how the Trust behaved, what else were they hiding from me?

All this would eventually be revealed. And it would turn out to be far more serious than anything I could ever have guessed.

Chapter 10 - Fielding and the Police

It was now January 2011. I had started to spend more time with Carl, who I felt was one of the few people who really understood what I was going through. I talked to him about my involvement with Cumbria Police and my growing belief that what happened to Joshua and the situation at the Maternity Unit at FGH should be criminally investigated. I gave Carl the contact details for DCS Goulding and Carl agreed to write to him. At the same time I provided the police with updates including the 'NMC Shit' revelations.

A few days later I had an email from a DCI Doug Marshall, an officer from Cumbria Force's Major Investigations Team. The email said that DCS Goulding had asked DCI Marshall to attend the inquest into Joshua's death. Following the inquest the police would be in a position to decide whether a further investigation was necessary.

DCI Marshall subsequently made arrangements to meet with us at my house on the evening of January 20th.

In the meantime the preparations for the inquest continued. A date was yet to be confirmed and I understood from my solicitors that the Trust were being slow to provide some of the documentation that the Coroner had requested. In the early afternoon of January 20th my solicitors forwarded to me a document that the Trust had released at the request of the Coroner. It was entitled 'Review of Maternity Services in University Hospitals of Morecambe Bay NHS Trust', written by Professor Dame Pauline Fielding[2]. It was dated March 31st, 2010 with two later revisions, dated June 30th and August 6th, 2010.

I read this report with a deep sense of shock. It talked about five Serious Untoward Incidents at Furness General in 2008, one of which it referred to as 'Baby T', which I knew must have been Joshua.

The report went on to describe a number of issues that seemed to be very serious indeed.

The unit in Barrow in Furness (FGH) has been the site of the cluster of a number of adverse outcomes...

It was clear from most of our interviews that team working is dysfunctional in some parts of the maternity service...

The legacy of the Serious Untoward Incidents has not helped here – the review team heard that relationships between obstetricians and paediatricians at FGH is improving but there is still much more that needs to be done...

The review team felt that multidisciplinary ward rounds do not take place on the labour ward at FGH.

The hospital facilities are not entirely fit for purpose, particularly

---

[2] I later learned that the Fielding Report had been commissioned by the Trust at the request of the North West Strategic Health Authority (NWSHA) in 2009, following concerns they had about the number of Serious Untoward Incidents at Furness General.

with respect to the labour ward environment and the distance of theatres and compare unfavourably with others in the Trust...

There is also a history of poor relationships between midwifes and neonatal staff although this was felt to be improving...

It became apparent during the course of the interviews that there is little understanding of the concept of clinical governance.

Training opportunities for midwifes are seen to be somewhat problematic with training budgets cut.

It was apparent during most of the interviews that there is a lack of common understanding of the role of the Supervisor at all levels of the organisation. This matter has a troubled history in the events which followed the SUI of Baby T [Joshua] but is not entirely related to this incident.

It was evident that the relationship between midwifes and senior managers had been damaged by the fallout from the incident but that this was gradually improving with some trust being restored.

The Trust has found it increasingly difficult to attract and appoint high calibre staff of all types. The staff working at FGH have found conditions to be challenging in the last few years.

For these reasons the morale of the staff in the maternity service has been badly affected. Relations between different categories of staff and between management have suffered within an atmosphere which at times may have embodied a 'blame culture'.

This was a recent report - these seemed like serious ongoing issues long after Joshua's death. Not only were they serious, they were central to what had happened to Joshua and the other cases I now knew about: 'poor relationships between midwives and neonatal staff' and 'dysfunctional' teamwork.

We still didn't know the identity of the doctor who the midwives claimed was bleeped and spoken to. Reading this made me angry but, more than anything else, very concerned that mothers and babies might be still at risk, despite all the time that had passed since Joshua died.

If the same issues that had contributed to Joshua's preventable death were still occurring, wasn't this a serious matter of ongoing public safety?

I had a lot on my mind that day. I was due to meet with DCI Marshall that evening and I knew that my meeting with him would be important.

As arranged, DCI Marshall arrived at my house in the early evening. My dad and Hoa joined us.

I talked through the sequence of events: what had happened to Joshua and what had happened since, right up to the Fielding Report that I had only received a few hours earlier. It was a lot of information, but DCI Marshall listened intently. We had a long and open conversation, of the kind I had become used to having with people in positions of authority. Only this was different.

At the parts which I had got used to being met with a look as if to say '…this guy's a grieving dad who's exaggerating', it was clear that there was genuine concern. DCI Marshall was to become another person who would significantly affect the story of our struggle to get to the truth.

The meeting finished on a positive note. I was to follow it up by forwarding some of the documents I'd referred to in our discussions. The fact that a senior detective was now going to attend Joshua's inquest could only be positive. There was something about DCI Marshall that instilled confidence.

The next day I thought that it might be a sensible move to pass a copy of the Fielding Report to the CQC. I assumed it was a document they would have been well aware of. What did they think about it? I sent an email to the Regional Director.

To my astonishment I soon learned that the CQC had never seen the report before.

My email to the Regional Director was the first time that the CQC had set eyes on the Fielding Report. I later learned that Monitor hadn't seen the report either, yet just months before, the Trust had been awarded Foundation Trust status.

I read the Fielding Report again: five Serious Untoward Incidents at the Maternity Unit at FGH in 2008. I remembered the initial meeting at our home with Halsall shortly after Joshua's death when I had asked if other babies had recently come to harm; the awkward pause followed by the carefully worded answer.

I thought back to the meeting I had with Halsall back in May a year ago. I still had the recording of this meeting on my phone. I played it back to double check I had remembered everything accurately.

I listened to the words again.

Halsall talked about the close scrutiny of the CQC. He then clearly stated:

There is nothing the CQC don't know about our organisation, or that we have not shared with them completely and openly.

During that meeting Halsall must have been well aware of the Fielding Report.

The Ombudsman had refused to investigate Joshua's death because they said the CQC was the appropriate body to ensure improvements were made - the Foundation Trust application was supposed to be a lever that would ensure that those improvements would happen.

How could it be right that the Trust was granted Foundation Trust status and yet neither the CQC nor Monitor had seen this damning report?

In the following days I discussed the Fielding Report with my solicitors and I mentioned that I had emailed a copy to the CQC. To my surprise, they took this extremely seriously. It was explained to me that the Fielding Report had been released as part of the inquest proceedings and that there were strict legal protocols about sharing such information. I subsequently emailed the Regional Director of the CQC and asked them to ensure that my disclosure was kept confidential. I was reassured they would.

Given that my solicitors had agreed to provide representation during the inquest free of charge, I certainly did not want to do anything that could jeopardise their support. For the time being I would have to keep the Fielding Report and the evidence of Halsall's apparent dishonesty confidential.

However, this recent development and the 'NMC Shit' email had changed my view of Halsall completely.

On February 25th Farrar, the Chief Executive of the NWSHA, finally responded to my request to undertake a proper supervisory investigation regarding the events that led to Joshua's death. Although he now acknowledged that the original LSA report was flawed in several respects, he refused to undertake the proper investigation I was asking for. Farrar gave various excuses in the letter, the main one being that the matter was now with the NMC. This was a very disappointing response.

After all this time there had still been no proper investigation into the circumstances of Joshua's death. The Trust's investigation was based on statements that I knew were not fully truthful and which hadn't even involved interviews with the staff. The supervisory investigation had been a complete whitewash. Wasn't it important for the safety of other mums and babies that a proper investigation was carried out as soon as possible?

On March 9th I sent a detailed letter of complaint about Farrar's decision and the supervisory process followed in Joshua's case to the Ombudsman. My letter drew attention to the other incidents I knew about and the apparent similarities. I wanted the Ombudsman to look at the governance of the NWSHA and ensure that lessons were learned from what were clearly major mistakes in Joshua's case. Unless this was done, other lives would be put at risk.

In late March I made contact for the first time with the parents of baby Alex Davey-Brady, Liza and Simon. I had read about their tragic case in the local paper after their inquest. I met with them both and was truly shocked by what they told me.

Alex Davey-Brady was born in Furness General Hospital on September 6th, 2008 – just seven weeks before Joshua was born. Baby Alex was tragically stillborn after the cord became trapped around his neck during a long and difficult birth[3]. Liza described failures in care that sounded terribly

---

[3] Liza and her partner's story, in their own words, can be found in Appendix 1

familiar. There was poor communication, Liza's concerns weren't listened to and there appeared to be a failure to involve doctors when help was needed.

Liza and Simon provided huge help and support to me personally and played a significant role in helping to uncover the truth that would eventually emerge.

Liza shared with me some key documents, including a copy of the expert medical report which was prepared for the inquest into Alex's tragic death. Liza also showed me another document that was to prove hugely significant.

This was a letter from a Dr Misra which was revealed as evidence at the inquest. It was written on October 17th, 2008 - just 10 days before Joshua was born.

Key extracts from Dr Misra's letter are as follows:

After going through the complaint made by the father, I have grave concerns about the management of this particular lady...

According to the father, it seems that Dr Surrey had taken 15-20 mins to attend and as soon as he entered the room he did not examine [the mother] or make any decision regarding possible Caesarean section. I have asked this question to Dr Surrey as this was one of the main complaints to me after the unfortunate incident. Dr Surrey replied that when he entered the room he was told by the attending midwife that the head had come down and everything was fine and normal and that he does not have to interfere or intervene at this stage. Obviously he waited outside the nursing station.

My main concern is that of trying to make every labour and delivery normal and natural and not thinking laterally [about] the possible complications.

113

Obviously this baby had died sometime in the second stage…

This has happened in our unit in the past and I am sure if we don't take appropriate precautions and positive steps, I am sure that this is going to happen again in future.

I had several thoughts when I read the letter. The first was that the events described suggested a situation whereby the midwives and the doctors were not working properly together.

The second thought was just how close to Joshua's birth this letter was written: just 10 days before. If the relationships between the doctors and the midwives were previously strained, what were they going to be like after the midwives became aware of Dr Misra's letter? How poor were relationships between the doctors and midwives at the time Joshua was born and how much did this influence the events that led to my son's death?

Finally I reflected on the words: 'This has happened in our Unit in the past and I am sure if we don't take appropriate precautions and positive steps, I am sure that this is going to happen again in future'.

This suggested that yet another preventable death at FGH had occurred. I thought of the poor family that this must have affected. Who were they and how long ago did this happen? I would later discover the answer and it was more shocking than I ever could have imagined.

Chapter 11 - The Inquest

On March 30th I got some very good news from DCI Marshall by email – the Cumbria Police were entering 'a formal investigation phase', researching and scoping the evidence and liaising with the Crown Prosecution Service. They asked me to keep my conversations with them confidential so as not to 'prejudice the investigation or cause any unnecessary alarm to members of the public'.

This was very significant news. I began to feel much better about the situation now the police were formally involved.

In early May I had a meeting with the CQC where they told me they would be attending the inquest. The CQC seemed to be more concerned about the situation at the Trust now that they were aware of the Fielding Report.

The dates were confirmed for the inquest: it would start on Thursday June 2nd, running though to Friday with a reserve date of Monday 6th if needed.

That month we took a three-week holiday at Disneyland in Florida. The plan was to spend time with the girls and get away from the mounting pressure. Although I tried my best, there were times when all I could think about was Joshua. He should have been coming to Disneyland with us - he would have been at the perfect age. These moments of sadness were now part of our lives. Nothing we could do would ever take them away.

The holiday finished just a couple of weeks before Joshua's inquest was due to start.

When we got back to the UK I could think of nothing else. Time went by very quickly and, before I knew it, Thursday, June 2nd had arrived.

On the morning of the inquest I met with my solicitor and the barrister about an hour before the start. They had a deep understanding of the issues involved in Joshua's case. This was immediately reassuring. My barrister, Paula Sparks, was very sharp. She was able to make sense of very complex information quickly and identify and focus on the key issues.

The inquest was held in a stately room in Barrow Town Hall. There were quite a few journalists present including TV and both local and national press.

Hoa and my dad were with me. I was concerned for Hoa. I knew that the next few days were going to be hard for us all but especially for Hoa, who still found talking about Joshua painful. It was for me too.

Day one of the inquest began with the Coroner giving an introduction and going over the formalities of the process. Hoa was the first witness called. She answered the questions clearly and calmly, going over everything that had happened in detail. The pregnancy, the birth, her collapse, her concern for Joshua, calling the bell by her bed in the early hours of the morning because she was so concerned about Joshua's breathing and the grunting sounds he was making and, finally, the moment early in the hours of Tuesday October 28th when she found him in a collapsed state in his cot and called for help.

Hoa finished giving her evidence with a broken voice and tears streaming down her face. It was awful to watch her relive her pain, but I felt so proud of her.

I was called to give evidence next. The Coroner went through the sequence of events in some detail. I had spent so much of the last few years of my life reliving the moments of Joshua's life and death that I did not find the process difficult at all. I gave my evidence clearly and with little emotion. It felt good being able to speak the truth.

Over the next two days we sat through the inquest as the Coroner interviewed the doctors, midwives and management staff about the circumstances of Joshua's death.

Much of what we heard was not the truth. At one point I had to leave the room as a midwife described the use of the overhead heater, stating that this was never placed over Joshua but was merely placed in the room. The two midwives who delivered Joshua described his birth exactly as they had done in their statements and not as Hoa and I remembered. This was very hard for us to hear.

The doctors were cross-examined in detail about whether or not they had received a bleep and if they gave advice to the midwives to monitor Joshua. All the doctors firmly refuted that they had ever received such a call, yet three midwives gave evidence that a call and conversation with a male doctor had taken place.

The Coroner also focused on the relationship between the doctors and midwives. The Trust's Maternity Risk Manager described the relationships in the Unit as 'dysfunctional' and 'strained'. However, the doctors and midwives said relationships were good. All the doctors called as witnesses started by offering their condolences to myself and Hoa. Not a single midwife even acknowledged us in the room. The atmosphere was hostile and defensive. It made me feel as if I was the one who had done something wrong.

As each midwife was interviewed the Coroner asked whether or not they were aware that a low temperature in a neonate was a possible sign of infection. Without hesitation, each and every midwife stated they were not aware that this was the case and that this had not been part of their training.

The Trust's barrister went on to argue that there was a 'national problem' at the time of Joshua's birth and that understanding the link between low temperature and possible neonatal sepsis was a widespread issue. When the Coroner had finished his questions my barrister questioned her with great skill, teasing out the inconsistencies. I looked around the room and I suspected that the representatives from CQC and the police were aghast at what they were hearing as the evidence unfolded.

However, my hopes that witnesses giving evidence under oath would lead to clarification of the many discrepancies about Joshua's life and death were quickly dashed.

On Friday 3rd it was clear that another day was needed and the Coroner announced that proceedings would finish on the following Monday. That evening Joshua's inquest was covered extensively on regional TV news and the next day it was the headline in the local paper.

On Monday the morning session heard evidence from Halsall himself who gave a convincing account, saying that the Trust had accepted the failures in Joshua's case from an early stage and had done a huge amount to put things right. Halsall did not accept that relationships between the doctors and midwives were strained and, when asked about staffing levels, said he believed the Unit was sufficiently staffed on the day Joshua was born.

The evidence sessions finished around midday and the Coroner called a recess for a couple of hours to prepare for his summing up. Hoa, my dad, my solicitor, my barrister and I retired to a private room to wait. A few hours later we were called back into the room to hear the verdict.

The Coroner started by explaining some basic facts about the inquest process and acknowledging what he described as the 'appalling tragedy' of our loss of Joshua. He then stated, 'I think it may be appropriate to just say that two doctors did the same and acknowledged your loss.... It has to be said no other medical person did'.

He then described the medical cause of Joshua's death as 'a left lung haemorrhage, the cause of that is a necrotic lung and the cause of this is pneumococcal sepsis'.

He then went on to discuss the verdict:

I did consider the possibility of natural causes with neglect. I have not gone for that. Neglect is a gross failure to provide medical care, and I am going to put it in this manner: that this is not the Scribes and Pharisees walking past on the other side of the road ignoring somebody who needs help. The medical staff did look in on Joshua and his parents. They did take his temperature from time to time. It is just that they did not recognise the signs that they were seeing as being what it was, which is a signpost to something very important...

The verdict I am reaching is what is known as a narrative verdict, which is this: Joshua Titcombe died from natural causes following a number of missed opportunities to identify that he was ill and to provide him with appropriate treatment.

At this point my heart sank. The circumstances of Joshua's death were so preventable and his signs of sepsis were so obvious, the failure to treat him earlier at Furness General could not be described as anything other than negligent. If this wasn't a 'gross failure to provide basic medical care', what was? However, any concern that the inquest was going to be a whitewash was soon put to rest.

The Coroner talked through the sequence of events from when Hoa's waters broke to our first visit to the hospital. He addressed the first point of discrepancy between the reported accounts of events and the evidence Hoa and I gave: during our first visit to FGH we described Hoa feeling poorly and having a sore throat and headache.

I accept that they said that. I accept completely that they did, evidence that they gave was consistent... It was not rehearsed, it was genuine evidence... this is the first example of a failure to record fully and accurately what was said and what information was known.

He went on to describe Joshua's birth and Hoa's subsequent collapse and commented on the lack of 'lateral thinking' in terms of the implications for Joshua. He then discussed the evidence given that a midwife had a telephone conversation with a paediatrician about Joshua.

No doctor that we heard from in evidence has got any recollection whatsoever of a telephone conversation from Holly Parkinson of answering the bleep in that matter in relation to Joshua... Dr Taufik was at pains to explain that he did not take this call, he was not the recipient of it. He is very aggrieved by an accusation levelled at him that he has fallen short of his professional standards and I have to say I agree with him. I do not think for one minute he took that call.

The Coroner then went on the say that he believed that such a call might have taken place.

It is possible that anyone in the room at that time might have taken this bleep and it is possible that the switchboard rang the wrong person. We do not know. It is more likely to me that there was a very short, a very non-specific conversation between [the midwife] and whichever doctor it was to the effect that the doctor in question has genuinely forgotten that it ever took place.

To this day I remain unconvinced by this explanation. I have to accept that I may never know for sure what really happened.

The Coroner continued:

In the course of Joshua's time, that very brief call was the only reference to a doctor at any point, and I include in that the two visits to the hospital previously, the only point at which a doctor became involved was Joshua's collapse... I get the impression that doctors did not step on midwives' toes, did not come and look unless they were invited to do so by the midwives.

He went on to describe the rest of Joshua's time in the post-natal ward:

During this period baby Joshua was not feeding well. He was obviously not maintaining his temperature, all clear signs to [the doctor] of potential sepsis, but the midwives did not know that, they gave evidence to that effect.

What he said next led to gasps from the people in the room:

I have got to say that the evidence given by the midwives on that specific point was so consistent and so clear, not one of them had any suspicion that a low temperature in a baby could indicate sepsis. I have to say, I think they got together at some point earlier... and I honestly believe that they collaborated and decided that they are going to stick together on that point...

I find it absolutely inconceivable that nobody on the department knew that simple basic fact, which is in the textbooks, and which they ought to have learned in basic training.

What the Coroner then went on to say was even more critical:

I am going to deal now with the missing observation chart, this yellow document that was set up as a consequence of [the midwife's] albeit very brief chat with a doctor whose identity is not clear, that document has gone missing. The only evidence I have heard about it, in terms of its contents that is, is that Mrs Titcombe remembers two specific readings, 35.8 and 36.1 degree, and I have to say I completely accept that those readings were on the chart... I come back to what I said some time ago, although readings were being taken, they were not being taken to heart... they were not being acted upon, because those readings, either of them, should have triggered off a report to a paediatrician for some fairly urgent action, but that did not happen.

As for the document itself, this yellow card or sheet of paper, it seems to me that there are a number of possibilities, the first being that it never did get photocopied, and the original went to Manchester with the rest of the copied notes. I cannot see why that would have happened, but it is a theoretical possibility. If that had happened then it would firstly have stood out, because it was yellow and everything else is a photocopy, therefore white. Manchester have not lost anything else, they have passed on notes,

122

and they went with Joshua when he ended up in Newcastle. So, I cannot really see how we can say that Manchester is likely to have lost the single bit of paper that was yellow that contains this important information. The second alternative is that is was not photocopied and it stayed in Barrow, in which case what did happen to it, which I will come back to. The third possibility is that it was in fact photocopied, in which case both the original and the copy have mysteriously gone missing, which is hardly credible at all, because they would not have stayed in one place. One would have stayed at Barrow, one would have gone to Manchester. So, to say, well amazingly both have got lost, one at Barrow and one at Manchester, or later Newcastle, is just not credible.

So, if it did not get copied, but stayed in Barrow, then I have to say it is not beyond the bounds of possibility that it was destroyed, and if it was destroyed that could only have been done deliberately. This is a piece of information about healthcare, it is the records of a human being, and it could not accidentally be thought to be a worthless piece of paper and thrown into recycling, or the bin...so the possibility does exist that somebody deliberately got rid of it because they realized that it did contain information, i.e. the readings that really could not be defended on the basis of no action having been taken.

He concluded by saying the loss of Joshua's observation chart:

...leaves a very worrying mark of suspicion hanging over why it is not there.

I believe this important record of Joshua's care was deliberately destroyed following his collapse and subsequent death. This remains one of the hardest aspects of coming to terms with what happened to my son.

The Coroner went on to describe the days leading up to Joshua's death and the last moments of his life:

I do not want to say this to upset his parents, but he died a pretty horrible death. He did not succumb gently to an infection as you can do, he had nine days in this world, the first day just not very well, from that point onwards extremely unwell, and then subjected to several extremely invasive medical procedures, despite which he sadly died on 5 November at Newcastle. These are the very sad and somewhat appalling facts as I see them.

This was hard to hear. I held Hoa's hand and we listened to the Coroner's closing comments in tears.

There was a moment when the Coroner gave me an acknowledging look and said:

I really do get the impression the doctors went on to the ward by invitation, you could say by invitation only. I think the midwives ran the show.

This was the exact phase he had used following the inquest into the tragic death of baby Alex Davey-Brady. This, it appeared to me, was the Coroner's way of making it clear that his view was that Joshua's death was not an isolated event.

In his final comments the Coroner listed the failures:

There was a failure to listen to and understand what the family said, what their concerns were about their own illness and whether that might pass on to Joshua.

There was a failure to record fully, or indeed on some occasions, to record at all many of the factors which, if they had been considered together, might have led to a greater degree of suspicion amongst the midwives and a referral to a paediatrician.

There was a failure to understand the basic medical fact that a low temperature and/or failure to maintain a temperature can be a sign of infection in a neonate.

124

There was a failure to notice and act on signs in Joshua, which should have prompted suspicion of infection.

There was an absence of continuity of care pretty well throughout the whole period that Joshua was being seen by anybody from Furness General, and I include in that before the birth, when his mum went in.

Mrs Titcombe and Joshua were treated as two unrelated individuals, and thought was not given to the fact that if something was affecting Mrs Titcombe it might have a bearing on how Joshua was.

There was a failure to think laterally, a failure to think holistically, not just for each of them, but for the two as mother and baby.

There is a failure even now to acknowledge by some members of staff that the recordkeeping was inadequate.

There is a failure by pretty well the whole of the staff to acknowledge that midwives acted as one team and doctors acted as a separate team, when to an outside observer they should act as a single integrated team.

I think there was enormous pressure on the midwives on the unit, which the reverse of the coin states that perhaps they were understaffed, but certainly on that particular day there were not enough people around to do everything that was necessary.

...inadequate, by which I think I really mean 'no' training for the midwives on the Post-Natal Ward to carry out the type of observations that the midwives on Special Care Baby Unit had been used to doing.

As in Baby Alex Davey-Brady's case, the inquest closed with the Coroner announcing he would be writing a 'Rule 43' letter. It was something that the Trust would be required to respond to formally.

A short time after the inquest closed, Cumbria Police issued a press statement confirming their ongoing formal investigation into Joshua's death. The next day the inquest was covered extensively in the local and national press. The *Daily Mail* reported the story under the headline: *It was a cover up.*

I had mixed emotions. I was pleased that, finally, we had achieved a substantially more comprehensive account of the circumstances that led to Joshua's death. At the same time, I was angrier than ever about what had happened to my son. Critical records had gone missing and the Coroner made clear his view that key evidence provided by staff was not believable.

A large part of me had hoped that the inquest would be an 'end point'. I soon realised that this couldn't be the case so long as so much remained unresolved.

I knew that the inquest would trigger further action, but I could not have imagined how far reaching the implications were going to be.

Chapter 12 - Action at last
– and a backlash

The following days were very intense. There was a lot of coverage in the media and I needed time to make sense of everything that had happened. The day after the inquest I was contacted by another family who had lost a child at the FGH Maternity Unit. In this case, the death had occurred after Joshua's death and the circumstances described were desperately tragic. How many more cases were there?

Halsall had written his weekly public blog about Joshua's inquest, following what by now seemed to be his standard line: the Trust had admitted they failed Joshua from the outset.

In this case dedicated and experienced staff failed to recognise the significance of specific risk factors. They did not recognise that Joshua was a very ill baby until it was too late.

The blog made no mention of the significant failures the Coroner identified, the critical medical records that had gone missing, the discrepancies in the evidence compared to what we remembered, the staffing levels, lack of training, dysfunctional relationships nor the Coroner's comments about staff 'collaborating' over their evidence. The Fielding Report had raised very serious concerns yet it had not been shared outside the Trust until I distributed it myself.

Any trust I previously had in Halsall was further eroded.

A few days later, I received a copy of the Rule 43 letter. It was damning. It highlighted four key issues: Record Keeping, Team Working, Pressure of Work and Continuity of Care. I would have to wait a few weeks before Halsall's response to it became available.

On June 13th I received news from the Ombudsman about the complaint I had made about the NWSHA (North West Strategic Health Authority) and the supervisory investigation into Joshua's death. It came as no surprise that it was yet another refusal to investigate.

We have not seen that the other instances highlighted involve similarities in terms of clinical issues or personnel to those found in Joshua's care. We have seen evidence that the NWSHA/ NWLSA considered events and took action to investigate; also that it referred to the NMC on occasion. We have therefore not seen indication of maladministration in how the NWSHA has discharged its duties on the basis of the information provided.

The letter concluded:

I fully appreciate therefore that you may be disappointed by our decision about the NWSHA/NWSLA. However, I hope that I have clearly explained the reasons for it and that there may be some little reassurance for you that the events prior to Joshua's death would not have represented missed opportunities to prevent what occurred.

I would eventually learn that the Ombudsman had not, in fact, looked in detail at the other cases I had referred to. I later formally appealed this decision by requesting an internal review. Here again, I had no success.

The only way in which it is possible to challenge an Ombudsman decision after requesting at internal review is by a process known as Judicial Review. I researched how to go about this process and I submitted a 'letter before claim'. As a result of this the Ombudsman eventually overturned their decision and agreed to investigate my concerns about the NWSHA and midwifery supervision. The report they produced was to have major implications for the regulation of midwifery in the UK.

On June 23rd, Halsall responded to the Coroner's Rule 43 letter. It was very defensive.

We do not believe that in Joshua's case a lack of team working was a contributory factor.

This seemed incredible to me in the light of the Coroner's very clear and specific remarks.

In relation to staffing levels, Halsall wrote:

We accept that the Maternity Unit was extremely busy on the day of Joshua's birth. However, we had a system at the time enabling additional staff to be brought onto the wards to assist, where necessary, which happened on that day. It is not clear to us as a Trust whether staff were 'stretched beyond their ability to cope' on that day... the issues identified in Joshua's care were not, in our view, due to insufficient staffing.

At the conclusion of Joshua's inquest, it hadn't occurred to me that the Trust could choose to simply reject the Coroner's findings, yet this seemed to be what Halsall was doing.

I shared Halsall's letter with the CQC and it was clear from their response that they were not impressed. By this stage I was in regular contact with the North West Regional CQC who were looking closely at the Maternity Unit at Furness General. I knew that they were planning to carry out an unannounced inspection visit in response to issues identified at the inquest and in the Fielding Report.

I also emailed my local MP, John Woodcock. I wanted to raise the Fielding Report with him and the serious concerns I now had about the Trust's response to the inquest. He did not seem to be very interested in responding.

I also contacted the Health and Safety Executive (HSE). However, the HSE was still adamant that they would not investigate Joshua's case. In late August the Chief Executive of the HSE, Geoffrey Podger, wrote to confirm that this.

HSE deals with the major non-clinical risks to patients such as trips and falls, scaling, electrical safety etc; and with some aspects of risks that apply to both staff and patients alike, such as manual handling. I recognise that this is not the response you were hoping for. I can, however, assure you that the issues have been considered very carefully to ensure we have made the right decision.

In the meantime, the CQC were moving quickly. In early September they published a report following the unannounced inspection they had carried out at Furness General Maternity Unit shortly after the inquest. It was damning. It found that the Trust was failing to meet six essential standards, with three 'major' and three 'moderate' concerns. This report was covered widely in the local and national media. I gave some interviews on local TV and radio. How could the Trust be failing to meet 'essential standards' in maternity services so long after Joshua's death?

The following day Cumbria Police announced that their investigation into Joshua's death had been widened to cover a number of deaths that occurred after mothers and infants received care at the FGH Maternity Unit. They now had 15 officers working full-time on the case. This led to more local and national headlines.

A few days later the CQC confirmed that they had issued the Trust with a formal warning notice, a legal document that required the Trust to take urgent action. The CQC's press announcement stated that the failure of the Trust to make the necessary improvements could result in the CQC taking further action. It was reported widely in the press that, if the necessary improvements weren't made, the CQC could take further action including the possibility of closing the Unit down.

This wasn't helpful to our family. Barrow-in-Furness is a geographically isolated town. The nearest Maternity Unit to Barrow is the midwifery-led unit at Westmorland General Hospital in Kendal, followed by the consultant-led unit in Lancaster. Both units are at least forty minutes to an hour away along the A590, a road well known for congestion and temporary road works.

It is therefore not surprising that many local people become extremely concerned at the possibility of their local Maternity Unit being closed.

I became aware of a Facebook group called 'Save FGH Maternity Unit'. Some of the messages posted were very personally hostile toward me.

I have to say I have had a miscarriage and one of my children there and the whole time I couldn't fault them but as I mentioned once before these people who have been interviewed on tv have then had it confirmed on the report that they went on to have another child which was healthy – I find it totally hypocritical of them to do that and then try to close the Unit down and force other mums through the painstaking job of having to travel further afield and putting panic and upset through them – it's so unfair and extremely untactful and undiplomatic!!

There were many other similar examples. I was shocked and deeply upset by the comments. I had certainly done everything I could to highlight what had happened to Joshua, but I had only ever done so out of a concern to ensure that the right lessons were learned so that no other parents would have to suffer a tragedy like ours.

The last thing I wanted was for the Maternity Unit at FGH to close - I just wanted it to provide a safe service.

More hostile comments began to appear in the on-line comments in the local paper:

I wonder if these rumours would have happened if the "minority" where white British children or mothers? My 2 kids where born at FGH and I couldn't fault them. I can personally understand how hard it is too lose close loved ones but not so early on in there lives. There is over 700,000+ babies born roughly each year and I for one think that the NHS is the best thing this country has.

Again, given that Hoa is from Vietnam, I couldn't help feeling that this was directed at me. Comments like this were something that I was going to have to get used to. But after struggling hard for so long, against the odds, to try and find out why my son died and how to prevent other similar deaths, to be cast now as a hypocrite and a troublemaker acting against the interests of other parents was something that was very hard to take.

In mid-September I had an update from the Nursing and Midwifery Council (NMC). The NMC had previously told me that their investigation into the midwives involved in Joshua's care had been put on hold pending the inquest. Now they were telling me that the NMC processes were on hold pending the police investigation.

I knew that the police investigation was likely to continue for some time, possibly years. The police investigation was looking at possible serious criminal issues. Surely the NMC, as the professional regulator, had a duty to look at the professional standards associated with what happened without any unnecessary delay? The NMC's decision not to progress their investigation felt wrong, especially given that the Strategic Health Authority had acknowledged that the supervisory investigation into Joshua's case had been flawed and that Mike Farrar, Chief Executive of the NWSHA, had pointed to the NMC as a reason for not carrying out another local investigation.

Towards the end of September my local MP, John Woodcock, published a letter that he had written to the then Secretary of State for Health, Andrew Lansley. John referred to the CQC report and how the Trust failed six 'essential standards' leading to Monitor giving the Trust a second 'red warning'. He then went on to say:

The vast majority of parents using the maternity unit are happy with the care they receive and that, whilst it is important that the issues raised by the CQC report and police probe are dealt with thoroughly, they should remain confident about attending the unit. I hope that if you or a member of your ministerial team do have the opportunity to do so, you would be able to give a similar message.

He ended the letter by seeking reassurance that the recommendations of the CQC report would be implemented as speedily as possible and that there would be no threat to the maternity service at Furness General Hospital.

The letter was unhelpful and insensitive. I could understand that John had a duty to represent the legitimate concerns of the local community regarding the future of services at Furness General, but wasn't it clear now that this was also about a service where lives had been put at risk and lost?

John wrote '...this is a very difficult time for the staff at Furness General Hospital, but also for the families who use the Maternity Unit there'. What about the families who, like us, had lost children? John knew about the Fielding Report which had not been shared with the regulators until months after. Why was he not making a noise about these issues or speaking up for other families who had lost loved ones?

I sent John a strong email making all these points.

On October 11th, 2011 Monitor announced that they had found the Trust in 'significant breach' of its terms of authorisation. The specific breaches were as follows:

(a) Condition 2: the general duty to exercise its functions effectively, efficiently and economically

(b) Condition 5: its governance duty

(c) Condition 6: its healthcare targets and other standards duty

The announcement from Monitor was published on their website with a detailed decision matrix setting out the evidence and the reasons for the action they were taking. This included the following:

The Trust has recorded two recent incidents on 27 and 28 September 2011, one in maternity involving the intrapartum death of a baby...The maternity incident appears to provide evidence of a midwife not appropriately involving medical staff or following guidelines, in a way that is a further and recent example of long-standing concerns.

I read this with some shock, a 'midwife not appropriately involving medical staff', just like Joshua's case. Yet another death. Just how much worse could the situation get?

Monitor announced that it was using its formal powers of intervention to require the Trust to 'accept the appointment by Monitor of independent external advisers to review maternity services and their interface with paediatrics... and to commission an independent review into overall governance including the Trust's approach to quality governance'.

In late October, yet more worrying news emerged. The 2011 Dr Foster Mortality Statistics for the Morecambe Bay Trust were announced. They were 124 - the highest mortality rate of any Trust in the country.

In the press the Trust claimed that these figures were not accurate, that the Trust's mortality ratio had not risen and the problem was to do with the way that the data had been collected.

Major problems were also reported with the Trust's outpatients appointments system. It was reported that a significant number of patients had not received outpatients appointments due to IT problems.

These issues, together with the recent CQC inspection report, the major criminal investigation by Cumbria Police and the recent intervention by Monitor led to mounting criticism of the Trust's leadership in the media.

The *Westmorland Gazette*, a local weekly newspaper, ran a number of hard-hitting headlines. In mid-October they published a statement from an anonymous 'whistleblowing consultant' from the Trust.

We have here a lame duck management with no credibility. I don't think there is any respect left for them among the clinical staff. Their inclination is to try to hang on to their jobs. A big fear is that Monitor will move in.

There is far too much focus on empire building and not enough listening to clinical staff. They are obsessed with hitting targets and box ticking.

I would have thought Tony Halsall would be considering his position on the board. Under normal circumstances you would expect senior managers to do the decent thing and step aside, but there is no sign they will do so.

If the board is not prepared to step down, the Secretary of State for Health should intervene.

Management has irreparably lost the confidence of doctors and other clinical staff.

You could draw a parallel with the mid–Staffordshire hospital's management failings – the obsession with hitting targets rather than focusing on clinical care, low staff morale, cost cutting, inadequate staffing, bullying and intimidatory atmosphere, disengagement between managers and clinical staff etc.

I am speaking out because I want to see the trust run like it should be, with the focus on patients, but I want my identity kept secret because the NHS doesn't treat whistle blowers sympathetically and I fear reprisals or even the loss of my job.

However, I don't think I will be a lone voice.

The issues at Morecambe Bay Trust were now much wider than Joshua's death alone; they were also wider than the growing concerns about the safety of maternity services at Furness General Hospital. In the past I had felt that things were only happening because I'd being pushing so hard, but I now realised that a chain of events had begun. The concerns were no longer mine alone; I had no control over what was happening.

On January 17th, 2012 the CQC announced that it was going to carry out a special investigation into the Trust's emergency care pathway. Yet more external scrutiny of the Trust's problems.

I continued to contact John Woodcock MP throughout this time, but by now our relationship had broken down. His office made it clear to me that he was not willing even to meet. John's view of the situation would eventually change.

Over the years since Joshua's death I had been in regular contact with the organisation Sands (the Stillbirth and Neonatal Death Society) which had been so helpful in the early days. I had agreed for Joshua's story to be included as part of a report Sands were producing called *Preventing Babies' Deaths - what needs to be done.* Joshua's story was used to highlight the importance of high quality investigations following avoidable perinatal death - a major recommendation of the report. I had been invited to the launch of the report on January 18th in the House of Commons. I attended with Hoa. Before the launch I let John Woodcock know about the event and his office replied to say that John might meet me there.

The event itself was powerful and emotional. I heard some extremely moving talks, including from other bereaved parents. Dan Poulter MP also spoke movingly about the work Sands was doing. Dan would later become the Under-Secretary of State for Health and would play an important role in our search for the truth.

The day reinforced my view of just how important Sands' work was. The report was excellent and I was proud that Joshua's story had been included. As it happened, I did bump into John Woodcock. We had a brief and frank conversation. John explained that while so many external processes were going on it was difficult to see what more he could do.

During the day I took the opportunity to introduce myself to Anne Milton MP who spoke at the event. Anne was the Under Secretary of State for Health and I had a brief conversation with her about Morecambe Bay. She told me that the Department of Health were keeping the situation 'under daily review'.

Locally, people were asking the Trust some difficult questions. In late January Halsall attended a meeting with the local Health Scrutiny Committee of Cumbria County Council. The Chair of the committee questioned Halsall about the Fielding Report, asking why it hadn't been shared externally at an earlier point. In a report of the meeting published on February 1st in the local paper, Halsall was quoted as saying that the decision not to share the Fielding Report outside the Trust was 'an error of judgement'.

I had a recording of the meeting I had with Halsall in May 2010 in which he clearly told me that there was 'nothing the CQC don't know about our organisation, or that we have not shared with them completely and openly'. I believed that the non-disclosure of the Fielding Report had been quite deliberate.

The bad news about the Trust continued. On February 2nd the CQC announced that it was issuing a second legal 'warning notice' to the Trust, this time relating to staffing levels in A&E.

On February 6th, 2012 Monitor announced that it would be using its formal powers to intervene for a second time to strengthen the leadership of the Trust. This involved:

- *appointing Sir David Henshaw as interim Chair to drive the recovery of the Trust*

- *requiring the Trust to appoint a Turnaround Director, to be agreed with Monitor, to develop and deliver an effective recovery plan*

- *instructing the Trust to create a Programme Management Office to support the Turnaround Director in delivering the recovery plan*

- *requiring the Trust to appoint an interim Chief Operating Officer, to be agreed with Monitor, to run the day to day activities of the Trust across all its hospital site*

- *requiring the Trust to report regularly on its progress in implementing the required actions and on addressing Monitor's residual concerns.*

The following day Monitor published the three separate investigation reports on its website: the diagnostic review of maternity services, a report on the outpatient issues and a Trust governance review.

All three reports were very critical.

The report on the outpatient issues highlighted a number of serious failures, including poor governance and risk management.

The Governance Review found that 'governance processes and systems are inadequate and are below the standard that we would expect in an NHS Foundation Trust'.

However, the Maternity Services Review was most shocking of all. The report stated that the review team had identified 119 unaddressed risks and concluded 'overall there remain significant risks for the safety of mothers and babies particularly at Furness General Hospital'.

I was stunned by this news. After all the reassurances that the Trust had given about improvements in maternity services, how could it possibly be the case that there were *still* 'significant risks for the safety of mothers and babies'?

With this news and the intervention that Monitor had taken to appoint at Interim Chair and a Turnaround Director, I thought that Halsall's resignation would be imminent. However, it wasn't. I was incensed.

Throughout this time I was in regular contact with Carl Hendrickson and Liza Brady, who both had lost babies at the Furness General Maternity Unit (and, in Carl's case, his wife as well). We discussed the situation and decided to create an online petition calling for Halsall's resignation.

I also decided that I would make the recording of the meeting I had with Halsall in May 2010 public. I contacted BBC Radio Cumbria and gave the journalist a copy of the recording.

On February 10th, 2012 Radio Cumbria aired the story. It was a very well constructed piece. The reporter explained the background to the Fielding Report, what it said and why it was a significant document. Then, live on radio, the recording I had made of the meeting I had with Halsall back in May

2010 was played for all of Cumbria to hear. The quality wasn't great, but you could clearly hear Halsall saying the words 'there is nothing the CQC don't know about our organisation, or that we have not shared with them completely and openly'.

It was a damning piece.

Carl, Liza and I also decided that we would write a joint open letter to Halsall, which we sent to the local paper. The letter was published that Saturday along with a very supportive editorial.

Our families recognise that mistakes can happen, and that sometimes such mistakes can have tragic consequences. We believe however, that such circumstances should be met with openness and honesty. When innocent lives have been lost, there is no room for denial, complacency, spin or propaganda. The only acceptable response is to quickly establish what went wrong and for everyone involved to do what ever is necessary to ensure such tragic events do not happen again.

Our families have been united by tragedy, but we also share a common struggle to establish the full truth regarding what happened to our loved ones. Our grief has been prolonged as a result; issues which should have been addressed long ago, have been allowed to carry on for much too long.

The reports published by Monitor this week are deeply shocking. How can it be that after all this suffering and heartache, mothers and babies at FGH were still found to be at 'significant risk' as recently as December 2011?

These past years have taught our families that under your leadership, University Hospitals of Morecambe Bay is a trust that simply cannot be trusted. The loved ones we have lost, our families and the local community, deserve much more that this.

141

With heavy hearts, please understand that we have had enough. We call upon you to take proper responsibility for the ongoing failures and to tender your resignation with immediate effect.

On February 24th, 2012, Halsall announced his resignation.

Despite the progress made, these events had left me with a sense of shock; since Joshua's inquest in July 2011, so much had unravelled, and it went far beyond my own personal tragedy.

How could so many serious problems at the Trust have now emerged when, just months earlier, Monitor had granted the Trust Foundation status and CQC had given the Maternity Unit at FGH the all clear?

Chapter 13 – 'The Musketeers'

Carl, Liza and I started to spend more time talking together. This collaboration between the affected families continued to develop and proved to be of crucial importance. All three families were now aware that the police investigation involved them. We discussed our experiences of the Local Supervising Authority investigations.

In Carl's case, the LSA had not even undertaken an investigation following the death of his wife and son. In Liza's case, despite a letter from a consultant that had expressed grave concerns about her care, an investigation was not carried out until several months after baby Alex's death.

Liza and Carl decided to refer their experiences of the LSA process to the Ombudsman. At the same time, I researched how to go about a Judicial Review. The first step of the process was to write what was called a 'letter before claim'. I spent the next few weeks carefully constructing a letter using a template I found on the internet. I completed this and sent it to the Ombudsman a few weeks later.

Yet more evidence of the failures of the Maternity Unit came to light. The police had looked at the letter that Dr Misra had written following the tragic death of baby Alex

Davey-Brady. This letter was written just 10 days before Joshua's birth.

Crucially it stated:

This has happened in our unit in the past and I am sure if we don't take appropriate precautions and positive steps, I am sure that this is going to happen again in future

By chance, Liza had been in contact with the mother referred to in Dr Misra's letter. The police had told her that her daughter's death was also part of their investigation.

To my shock, this was the kind lady I had met in the local flower shop on the day of Joshua's funeral. She had been very upset when I explained the flowers I was buying were for the funeral of my baby boy. She told me about the death of her own daughter and said that it was 'just one of those things and there was nothing anybody could have done'.

Now, more than seven years later, this poor woman was confronted with the fact that her daughter's death was part of a major police investigation and the possibility that what she had been told by the Trust at the time was not the full truth.

In early March I finally had a formal meeting with John Woodcock MP.

Liza and her cousin came with me. It is fair to say that this was a truly awful meeting. John seemed distant and disinterested. We discussed all the issues which we felt John had not got right including his letter to Andrew Lansley, which had failed to mention the devastating impact the problems at the FGH had had on families who had lost loved ones. We asked why he had not done more to speak up for our families and to hold the Trust to account.

The tenor of the meeting did not improve. John said that he had no regrets and would not have done anything differently.

We left the meeting feeling frustrated and dejected.

In mid-March I had a meeting with Sir David Henshaw, the new Trust Chair who had been put in place by Monitor at Morecombe Bay. It was a frank conversation. Henshaw was clear that he wasn't there to defend past events and was appalled by what he had heard. The Trust was very concerned about the ongoing police investigation. Henshaw said that the Trust would like to do something to 'hold Joshua's name in memory' and asked me to think of ways in which this could be done.

After the meeting I emailed Henshaw to say that, although I appreciated the gesture, it wouldn't be fair to single out Joshua as so many other lives had been lost. The best way he could honour Joshua's memory and the other lives lost was to help establish the full truth.

On March 28th, 2012, I sent an email to Anne Milton, the Under Secretary of State for Health I had met at the Sands event, calling for a full Public Inquiry. I copied in MPs John Woodcock and Tim Farron.

I followed this up with an email to John Woodcock asking if he would support my call for an inquiry. John replied saying 'I am not convinced at this stage that a public inquiry would be appropriate in addition to the various other investigations, but will keep this under review'.

Around the same time, the *Health Service Journal* (HSJ) published a piece about a review Monitor had conducted into the decision to grant Morecambe Bay Foundation status in 2010. The article included the following:

Monitor's executive chair has admitted it is 'very likely' University Hospitals of Morecambe Bay had 'deep-seated problems' at the time his organisation granted the Trust foundation status.

David Bennett [the Chief Executive of Monitor] told the HSJ that 'the regulator needed to further toughen its assessment process after major failings in the Trust's management and maternity services came to light within 12 months of its authorisation'.

Mr Bennett told the HSJ: 'I accept that it's very possible, very likely even, that there were issues – deeper issues – at the time of assessment.

'The regulator said it would introduce a detailed "quality governance" assessment for applicants, to ensure, in part, that they were identifying and managing care quality risks, and taking action on substandard performance'.

But asked if Monitor had applied these checks at Morecambe Bay, Mr Bennett replied: 'The simple answer is no'.

The CQC was also quoted in the piece:

CQC director of operations Amanda Sherlock said she now believed there were underlying problems at Morecambe Bay in 2010.

'If the provider isn't able to identify risk and take steps to mitigate those risks it is unlikely to be able to respond proactively to developing concerns, and I think that would be our view of where Morecambe Bay was at,' she said. 'It didn't know what it didn't know'.

She acknowledged that, as with Mid Staffordshire, the drive for foundation status could have been 'a distraction' for the

Morecambe Bay board 'when they should have been focusing on core elements of the quality of their services'. But since April 2010 'ourselves and Monitor are always mindful of understanding where there may be an over-focus on the attainment of foundation trust status'.

I thought about this article a lot, especially the words 'it didn't know what it didn't know'. What did this statement actually mean? Certainly, the CQC and Monitor were aware of serious concerns with maternity services at FGH as early as 2009. In December that year the Regional Director of the CQC had sent me a letter that included the statement:

I am able to confirm that at the present time we have a number of concerns about the operation of UHMBT, some of which stem from information the Trust has provided to us about its own investigations surrounding Joshua's death and some of which are quite separate.

The letter had even warned of 'future tragedies' if improvements weren't made.

We believe that if future tragedies are to be avoided, the Trust needs to be able to evidence a much more integrated approach to care.

I also knew that the concerns CQC had about the Trust at this time had led to Monitor suspending the initial Foundation Trust application.

In terms of what the Trust itself knew, in March 2010 Halsall was in possession of the Fielding Report. The issues that the Fielding Report identified did not seem significantly different to those now being discussed. What exactly *didn't* the Trust, CQC or Monitor know?

For me, this article raised further questions: if such clear concerns were widely held at the end of 2009, what processes did the CQC and Monitor then go through to assure themselves that the problems had been addressed?

On March 30th, 2012 an article appeared in the *Daily Telegraph* with the headline *Health regulator 'still failing' in duty to protect patients.* The piece focused on comments that Kay Sheldon, a non-Executive Director at the CQC, had made about the regulator, including the actions taken at Morecambe Bay.

In the piece Kay is quoted as saying:

'The culture is oppressive and there have been allegations of bullying that have not been investigated. The organisation is in crisis mode and is still concerned with its own reputation.'

She said inspectors had failed to detect risks to patients at Furness General Hospital, in Barrow, where seven babies died and only took the issues seriously after the coroner intervened.

Ms Sheldon said she raised concerns about the quality of the CQC inspections and the lack of action taken with the CQC board but was told it had been a 'robust' piece of work.

'I am concerned that we are not an effective regulator of health and social care.

For example, I have serious concerns about how effective the CQC was in identifying and acting on concerns at Morecambe Bay hospital trust in the maternity services...

The inspectors are not specialists in their areas and have heavy workloads so even when they did identify risks to patients those were not followed up on by the CQC.

It is only when Monitor and the coroner identified the same and more serious problems that the CQC began to take the issue seriously.'

Tim Farron, the Liberal Democrat MP for Westmorland and Lonsdale, was certainly taking the issues seriously.

On May 12th the *Westmorland Gazette* published a piece under the headline: *Morecambe Bay maternity problems 'may have been overlooked by health watchdog', claims MP.*

The article reported MP Tim Farron's concerns that in June 2010, almost two years after Joshua's death, the CQC found the Maternity Unit at FGH fully satisfactory yet in December 2011, following Joshua's inquest, Monitor found 119 risks.

'This is extremely concerning news and raises a whole new question as to whether we should be investigating the regulators...' said Farron. 'I will now be seeking reassurances from both the Health Secretary and the CQC that the failings in the model for inspection are being reviewed and corrected in order to prevent further disasters like the crisis at UHMBT'.

In mid-April 2012 the Trust finally provided me with 3 large folders of information that I had requested under the Data Protection Act (DPA) following the discovery of the 'NMC Shit' email.

These documents were extremely troubling.

On April 19th, 2009, the day after Joshua's story had been published in the local paper, an email from the Trust Maternity Risk Manager (also the author of the LSA report into Joshua's death) to the Trust's Customer Services Manager included the following:

The local press coverage was even worse than I anticipated and I new it would be bad. 3 page spread and in my opinion mostly about James! There you go – I am a nasty person.

Have spent the last few days stopping the staff from committing Hari Kari – one gone off sick

Happy days! Hope you are OK

As I keep saying to the girls we will get through this together Muskateers!

There was another email dated June 2nd, 2009 from Halsall to the then Chair of the Trust. The email was titled 'Mr T'.

Good morning [to the former Trust Chair],

Sorry my battery did die and I then got stuck in the airport transfer etc.

I have attached an email for information just as an update on the JT issue. He is furious about a discrepancy of 0.4 of one degree in the baby's temp but as we have discussed this is all predictable in terms of fighting with the detail.

*I will be speaking again with Miranda but after I speak with the CQC again as I think they have now done what they told me they were doing in terms of the SHA team etc. As soon as I know what they are saying to Monitor I will then push at Miranda. I am going to suggest that you and I go and pay them a visit with Peter and June which I think they will go with. **If I'm correct then the CQC can cover off the Ombudsman in their response if they are prepared to have that conversation with them which they didn't indicate they were not.*** [my bold]

In June 2009 the Ombudsman had been considering my request to investigate Joshua's death for some time. What did Halsall mean by 'If I'm correct then the CQC can cover off the Ombudsman in their response'?

I was very troubled by this. When the Ombudsman eventually refused to investigate Joshua's death, one of the main reasons given to me was that the CQC would ensure standards at the Trust improved. The subsequent reports by Monitor clearly showed that such improvements had not taken place. What did Halsall mean by '...if they are prepared to have that conversation with them which they didn't indicate they were not?' What conversations had taken place between the CQC and the Ombudsman prior to their decision not to investigate Joshua's death?

I had to find out.

There was further cause for concern.

A document titled *Inquest – Joshua Titcombe Q&As* was dated June 1st, 2011, a few days before Joshua's inquest. It was structured under a number of different headings including Infection, Care of Joshua, Factual Disputes, Joined Up Care, Care Post Collapse. Under each section were questions or statements about Joshua's care with 'answers' written beneath each one.

What was the purpose of this document? Who had written it? Had the content been shared with staff before Joshua's inquest?

The document read like a transcript of the evidence given at the inquest.

It included statements like 'There was a lack of awareness by the staff that persistent hypothermia in the neonate can indicate sepsis' and 'There was a lack of recognition by the staff of the relevance of neonatal hypothermia and the need to refer for a medical assessment. It stated:

The midwives who cared for Joshua trained and worked at different Trusts, in addition to FGH, and during their training, the prevention, management and consequences of neonatal hypothermia focussed on achieving normothermia by maintaining a warm environment, warm hat and clothes and promoting early feeding.

These were all themes that emerged in the evidence of the midwives in response to questions asked by the Coroner and the Trust's barrister.

I made a request to the Ombudsman for all information they held (under DPA) and wrote to the Trust to ask for an explanation regarding the Q&A document. This would eventually reveal even more disturbing material.

Chapter 14 – News from the Ombudsman

In May 2012 I had some unexpected news from the Ombudsman.

Following the 'letter before claim' I had written a few months earlier, the Ombudsman had carried out a second external review of their decision not to investigate my complaint about the LSA investigation into Joshua's death, concluding that their decision not to investigate 'did not stand up to scrutiny'.

It was a well-written review, logical and very clear. As a consequence, the Ombudsman had agreed to reassess my complaint from scratch. The Ombudsman was now formally considering Carl and Liza's complaints too.

My first complaint to the Ombudsman in April 2009 had included my serious concerns about the supervisory investigation and the LSA's response to Joshua's death. When the Ombudsman refused to investigate, I was advised to raise my complaint with the North West Strategic Health Authority. I pursued this only to be told that the supervisory investigation into Joshua's death was 'commendable'. Only after involving the Nursing and Midwifery Council did a second review find that, in fact, the supervisory investigation was 'flawed'. Even with this admission, the NWSHA refused to undertake a proper supervisory investigation.

I had then complained formally to the Ombudsman only to have my complaint rejected. I had gone through the appeal process and my complaint had been rejected once again. It was only now, after doing my own research on how to go about a Judicial Review and starting the process, that the Ombudsman was finally acknowledging their previous decision was flawed. I wondered how many people in similar situations to me had been defeated by the seemingly endless obstacles put in their way.

The *Health Service Journal* covered the story on May 24th, 2012, reporting that the Ombudsman's own review into the rejection of my complaint 'appeared to be directly contradicted by its own documents'. The article then went on to report how the Ombudsman had originally denied any similarities with the other cases I had raised with them the previous June but later admitted 'we have not looked at the investigations themselves because they are about other cases'. It quoted my comments on the contradictions of the Ombudsman's process – 'before they do an investigation they have to be satisfied of a 'worthwhile' outcome. How can you tell there will be a worthwhile outcome before you investigate?' – and my belief that if the Ombudsman had investigated my complaint in 2009, the whole series of events that unfolded at Furness General Hospital could have been avoided.

On the same day I received a letter from Stephen Dorrell MP, the Chair of the Health Select Committee, who I had written to previously about the Ombudsman's decision not to investigate Joshua's death.

154

*While I cannot comment on the way in which your case was han-
dled by the Ombudsman, it does seem to me unsatisfactory that
the regulatory actions and additional investigations to which you
refer were only undertaken in consequence of a Coroner's report
made for the purposes of preventing future deaths and not as a
consequence of any investigation carried out by the Ombudsman.*

This was significant. As the Chair of the HSC, Stephen
Dorrell had considerable influence and his dissatisfaction
with the Ombudsman's procedures was clear.

In late June I received a large number of documents from the
Ombudsman in response to my request under DPA. Among
the documents was a memo written by Kathryn Hudson, the
former deputy Ombudsman, to Ann Abraham, the current
Ombudsman. The memo was titled 'Note of telephone conversation with [the regional director of the CQC]' and was
dated the September 10th, 2009.

*In your conversation with Cynthia Bower [the former CEO
of the CQC] shortly before your leave, the suggestion arose that
if we could assure Mr and Mrs Titcombe that as a result of
their experiences CQC are now taking robust action to ensure
improvements in the quality of maternity services in the Trust,
you might decide not to investigate.*

The email Tony Halsall had written to the Trust Chair in
June 2009 included the words 'If I'm correct then the CQC
can cover off the Ombudsman in their response if they are
prepared to have that conversation with them which they
didn't indicate they were not'.

Why were the two most senior people at both the CQC
and the Ombudsman discussing my son's case in this way?
What did Tony Halsall mean by the phrase 'cover off'?
Was there some behind-the-scenes deal going on here,

155

the consequences of which were that the serious failings at Furness General continued long after Joshua's death?

It seemed scandalous. In the four years since Joshua had died every stone that I turned over revealed something deeply unpleasant or profoundly unjust.

I was more determined than ever to continue to push for answers until the full truth was established.

Chapter 15 – Campaign Mode

On July 13th, 2012 the CQC published its report on the investigation into the delivery of emergency care at the Trust which it had announced back in January.

It was yet another damning report. The CQC press release stated that '...patients remained at risk of poor care, particularly those in accident and emergency and other parts of the hospital that provided urgent care'.

Concerns remained about inconsistent incident reporting practices, lack of learning from incidents and poor use of performance information to drive change.

Despite all the previous reports and reviews, the serious problems at the Trust were continuing.

I was doing everything I could to draw attention to these issues. On July 15th, 2012 the *Sunday Post* covered Joshua's story and my calls for a public inquiry on the front page.

In July 2012 the Trust responded to a request I had made under the Freedom of Information Act about the number of cases of death or serious harm at the Maternity Unit at FGH which had resulted in legal action. The information provided was, once again, deeply shocking. I forwarded it to the local and national press.

Based on this information, the next day *The Guardian* reported that FGH faced more than 30 compensation claims over deaths of, or injuries to, mothers and babies and that the Trust had admitted there had been 37 civil claims[4] in all since 2002, only five of which had been settled, and 24 claims have been made since the start of 2011.

It quoted Tony Halsall as saying 'considerable progress' had been made on improving the position before he had resigned in February. Eric Morton, the interim CEO, apologised for the serious failings of their maternity services in the past and DCI Marshall of Cumbria Police confirmed that their 'full and thorough investigation' was continuing.

On July 19th I had a reply from the Department of Health following my email to Anne Milton.

The Department of Health has noted the issues you have raised about the care of your son and I understand that this continues to be a difficult time for you and your family. As I have explained in previous correspondence, it is not appropriate for Ministers or the Department to intervene in this matter.

The Department of Health were not yet supporting the inquiry calls - their position would eventually change.

I had made contact with Kay Sheldon, the CQC Board member who had expressed concerns about CQC's actions

---

[4] The Trust subsequently updated their response to my FOI request, stating that they had made an error and that the correct figures were 29 civil claims relating to incidents at FGH since 2002.

at Morecambe Bay in the *Daily Telegraph* article in March. I provided Kay with everything I had on the CQC's actions following Joshua's death and recent information about the scale of harm that had been taking place.

I was now in regular contact with Peter Walsh, the Chief Executive of Action against Medical Accidents (AvMA), who had been so helpful in providing advice and support in the early days after Joshua's death. Peter agreed that AvMA would formally support my calls for an inquiry into the events at the Trust.

In late July 2012 Peter set up an on-line petition and published an open letter to Andrew Lansley calling for an inquiry into events at the Trust. Peter also wrote to MPs Tim Farron and John Woodcock. The numbers of signatures on the petition grew and pressure began to mount.

Around this time, I also made contact with a journalist at *The Independent*, Nina Lakhani, who was very interested in the documents I had unearthed.

On July 30th, 2012 *The Independent* published a major story under the headline 'Watchdog waited two years to act over failing maternity units'.

Last night calls for an independent inquiry into the regulatory failings involving the trust – where thousands of outpatient appointments were 'lost', security guards stood in for nurses, patients were left unattended in A&E without pain relief for seven hours - intensified. The failures happened just months after the scandal at Mid Staffordshire came to light – which was also certified as safe and sound by regulators as people were dying needlessly from substandard care.

It was very critical of the whole CQC regulatory process, reporting that systematic failures at the Morecambe Bay

NHS were suspected by the CQC more than two years before it finally launched an investigation that exposed 'scandalously poor care'.

It pointed out that no trust had been judged to have failed by the CQC, yet serious concerns had emerged about several hospitals, including Basildon and Thurrock as well as Morecambe Bay. Importantly, it also referred to the email Tony Halsall had written to the Trust Chair in June 2009 which included the dubious phrase 'if I'm correct then the CQC can cover off the Ombudsman…'

The story included comments from John Woodcock and myself, questioning the CQC's claims that the Trust was fully compliant at the time of registration and that, since then, it had 'escalated its scrutiny of the Trust, taking enforcement action and carrying out an investigation'. Peter Walsh of AvMA emphasised the need for an independent inquiry and commented that the CQC were 'far too willing to accept unsubstantiated assurances and get cosy with the Trust rather than look beneath the surface'.

In the following months I wrote to the CQC to express my concerns. On August 31st I met Amanda Sherlock, the CQC's Director of Operations. We had a long conversation about how the CQC had acted. I had become so distrusting of all organisations involved in the NHS I recorded the meeting. I couldn't believe what Mrs Sherlock told me:

If the Ombudsman had decided to do an investigation into Joshua, that would have triggered concerns that we would have looked at as to the organisation's capacity and capability… If the Ombudsman had launched an investigation in 2009 we would have taken, I am certain, very different decisions.

This was alarming. The Ombudsman had told me that one of the reasons why they decided not to investigate Joshua's death was because they were satisfied the CQC's oversight of the Trust would ensure it made the necessary improvements. Now the CQC were telling me that the Ombudsman's decision had been taken as reassurance that everything was OK.

I could not understand how this could have been possible.

During this meeting Amanda Sherlock told me that the CQC were listening to the concerns and would be carrying out a review to investigate what happened and look to learn lessons.

In October I made a formal submission the CQC covering the issues that I wanted the investigation to consider. The review they commissioned became known as the Grant Thornton investigation and was to have significant implications.

In August 2012 the Trust supplied the documents I had requested under the Data Protection Act that hadn't already been provided.

I found an email chain that started back on June 10th, 2010 when I had emailed the Customer Care Manager to say I was extremely distressed and wanted to step back from my efforts and look after my family.

The same afternoon the Customer Care Manager had emailed the Head of Midwifery at the Trust. It said:

Good news to pass on re JT.

That evening, the Head of Midwifery replied:

Has JT moved to Thailand? What is the good news?

This was deeply upsetting. Hoa is from Vietnam not Thailand, but it was clear what the basis of comment was: a joke suggesting that it would be good news if my family and I went back to where my wife was from.

I emailed the Trust to raise these issues and eventually referred my complaint to the Ombudsman.

In November 2012 I met with the CQC's new Chief Executive, David Behan, at their offices in London. It was a helpful meeting. David clarified the current terms of reference for the CQC's review of Morecambe Bay. He confirmed that the terms covered the CQC's actions at the Trust from April 2010 to April 2012. During the meeting I explained the concerns I had over how the CQC acted prior to April 2010, particularly the response to Joshua's death, how it communicated with the Ombudsman and why the Trust's risk rating was de-escalated prior to it being registered without conditions. Following this meeting, the CQC confirmed that the Grant Thornton review had been extended to cover these earlier concerns. This was to be much more significant that I could have imagined at the time.

Around this time I also started to work with a TV Producer who was making a *Panorama* programme about the safety of the NHS. The film crew came up to Cumbria and interviewed me about what happened to Joshua and our experiences since.

I got more encouraging news from John Woodcock MP. John agreed to meet with me and Peter Walsh - a significant turning point in terms of John's support for our campaign. John signed the online petition and gave very supportive comments in the local paper. In November 2012 he also wrote to Jeremy Hunt to support calls for a fully independent inquiry and to request a meeting with him, along with myself and a representative from AvMA.

This was a very important development: our local MP was now formally writing to the Secretary of State in our support.

The momentum was building. Peter Walsh was helping to keep up the pressure and I was also in contact with Dr Kim Holt who had set up Patients First, an organisation which supported whistleblowers and campaigned for greater openness and transparency in the NHS. Patients First also strongly supported our call for an inquiry.

In early December the *Panorama* episode aired on BBC1. This had a big impact and added more force to our campaign for an inquiry.

By this time, I had made contact with the journalist Shaun Lintern who had played a key role in helping to uncover events at Mid-Staffordshire. He was a reporter for the local paper in Stafford and now worked for the *Health Service Journal (HSJ)*. Shaun was taking a huge personal interest in the events at Morecambe Bay and took the time to have long conversations with me to understand the details.

In December Shaun wrote a compelling piece in the *HSJ* highlighting the issues being investigated by the CQC external review.

In mid-December 2012 Cumbria Police issued a press release confirming that they would soon begin interviewing the staff involved at FGH. This was an important development: the police would not be investing the time and the resources needed to take the investigation forward unless there was a real chance of a prosecution.

In early January 2013 Carl, Liza and I started to discuss how we could take the campaign for an inquiry forward. I proposed that with all the information we now had, we could create a website and launch a formal campaign group. We found a website designer and Liza and I agreed to go halves on the cost.

We spent some time thinking about how the website would look and what we wanted it to say. We agreed to call the campaign group 'Morecambe Bay Inquiry Action'. Liza and Simon helped design a logo and we worked together on the content. We also set up a Facebook group.

On January 9th, 2013 I met with the new Parliamentary and Health Service Ombudsman, Dame Julie Mellor, in London. The meeting was to discuss the concerns I had about the Ombudsman's decision, taken back in 2010, not to investigate Joshua's death. The meeting went well and we agreed a way forward. Dame Julie confirmed that the Ombudsman would now formally investigate my complaint about the LSA investigation following Joshua's death.

The Ombudsman also proposed to carry out three additional investigations of the following issues:

1) How the Morecambe Bay Trust itself responded and investigated Joshua's death.

2) The evidence I had collected which raised serious concerns regarding the way in which the Trust and its staff had prepared itself prior to Joshua's inquest. Central to this was the document I had found, dated a few days before the inquest, which appeared to be a list of questions that the Coroner might ask together with model answers.

3) The email which contained a report about the circum- stances of Joshua's death, which a midwife had titled 'NMC Shit'.

I liaised with Ombudsman caseworkers as the investigations progressed over the months ahead.

In late January 2013 the Trust announced that, after the police investigation had concluded, they would be holding an internal inquiry into the past failures in their maternity services. Liza, Simon and I all felt strongly that the last thing we wanted was an internal review by the Trust. We needed a fully independent inquiry and we were determined to campaign for it.

We agreed to have an official launch of Morecambe Bay Inquiry Action (MBIA) on Wednesday January 30th, 2013. I sent an email to Sir David Henshaw, the Interim Chair of the Trust appointed by Monitor, to ask if anyone from the Trust wanted to attend.

He declined the invitation.

During the next few days Liza and I worked flat out on the website content. It covered the history of the problems and the timeline of events, as well as key documents and reports. The website went live on January 28th. Liza and I worked hard organising the launch day. We booked a venue in Barrow and I prepared leaflets and invited the local paper.

Around 10 different families attended the launch. It was a moving and emotional event. The local ITV News crew filmed the meeting and interviewed some of the families. The reporter from the local paper also took notes and interviewed people.

The event went well and the message was clear: all the families wanted to ensure that the truth was told so that lessons could be learned to prevent others suffering. I hoped the media coverage would raise the profile of the campaign, but this didn't happen. The following day the Trust made an announcement that overshadowed everything else.

Without any prior warning the Trust announced that, due to high sickness rates amongst staff at Furness General, it was transferring all consultancy-led maternity services to Lancaster Royal Infirmary. The announcement laid the blame for the high sickness and absence rates on the ongoing police investigation.

Within minutes of the news breaking some very upsetting messages appeared on the local paper's internet site:

i have been a midwife for 39 yrs the last 12 yrs i worked at fgh and they were the happiest days of my career until the last 3 yrs i have worked with a fantastic caring team ranging from the cleaners auxillaries maternity assistants and midwives and doctors .i have now retired so therefore im free to express my feelings .firstly i am so worried that this latest step will become permanent as we have been predicting over the last year yes the sickness levels amongst the staff are sky high at the moment blamed it seems from the trust statement on the police investigations as i am involved in this i can verify the treatment we are receiving is horrendous i felt like a criminal whilst being interviewed and never want to repeat this and secondly lack of support by the powers that be has to also have been a factor .you the lovely people of barrow deserve better stand up and be counted .i have a very heavy heart tonight and as the other person pointed out there are people in barrow whose sole aim has been to bring maternity sevices to their knees I HOPE THEYRE PROUD OF THEMSELVES"

Posted by linda on 31 January 2013 at 17:16

Well it was inevitable, well done to those of you who have been extremely vocal in your campaign against this unit, helped in no

*small part by the North West Evening Mail who appear inca-
pable of writing anything positive about the unit. Yes there have
been mistakes made, and these have led to tragic circumstances.
However, amongst those blissfully rare incidents are tales of
hundreds of births which have gone to plan with nothing going
wrong and tales of miracles being worked by the staff saving
lives. Sadly this doesn't make good news copy for the paper and the
don't get published. It is no wonder therefore that the midwives
and nurses that work on these units feel so under stress they are
having time off work, my heart goes to them.*

*I hope that this decision does not cause anyone harm and is a
temporary issue. If not then I know who I will blame and it will
not be the staff but the small vocal minority who live Ian world
where clearly nothing ever goes wrong and mistakes never made!*

Posted by Frustrated on 31 January 2013 at 16:32

*Bravo to those who have fought for this, your pursuit has ruined
more lives, but hey you got what you want at the expense of
thousands of people and the safety of them and their child, clap
clap clap*

Posted by Jeff on 31 January 2013 at 16:23

*Well done to those who have consistently pursued a vendetta
against the maternity unit. You know who you are. You succeeded
and the blood of innocents are now to be on your hands. Sickness
levels are high because of the enormous stress midwives and nurses
are under because of this endless battering. I hope you are proud.
Keep up the good work and eventually you will succeed in closing
your failure of a hospital. This is disgraceful*

Posted by Kira on 31 January 2013 at 15:21

The constant abuse of dedicated professionals has resulted in closure of emergency services to the most vulnerable members of the public. Temporary or not why has the Board not protected the very people needed to run this service. Unfortunately staff are not able to defend themselves publically and have been extremely brave for far too long. Each individual has a breaking point and because of this lives are now at risk.

Posted by pete on 31 January 2013 at 19:26

totally agree with Kira..the people baying for heads to roll now have certainly won... consultants heads have rolled to Lancaster.. well done..And yes i feel for the person who lost a dear beloved baby, but you obviously thought the trust were capable and in safe hands when your wife had another baby at FGH Maternity Centre!!.. Shocking Result… and yes I have had a child there in the last 5 years and my husband nearly lost me in childbirth but if it wasnt for the consultant i wouldbe be hear today..so some other poor woman may not be so lucky thanks to all the bad publicity, which has led to valuable and experience staff leaving, going on sickness leave..or no-one is applying for jobs thanks to your vendetta..

Posted by michelle on 1 February 2013 at 07:58

I was deeply shocked by the vitriol thrown at myself and Hoa. The idea that I was part of 'a vendetta' against the Maternity Unit when all the evidence suggested the midwives had colluded to protect themselves was outrageous and very hurtful. I just couldn't understand how, after years of struggle to get to the truth, I had become the guilty party, the one with 'blood on my hands' and who had 'ruined more lives'. It was very hard to take.

168

The other families I was in touch with felt the same. I had never wanted the Maternity Unit at FGH to close or be downgraded. All I wanted was to establish the truth about my son's death and for all the lessons to be learned to prevent other people suffering as we had.

The next day I read that there was going to be an emergency meeting in Barrow to discuss the situation for those concerned about the news. Despite the likelihood of a hostile reception I decided to attend and do my utmost to get my message across.

The meeting was in a local infant school. John Woodcock was answering questions when I arrived. The anger and concern in the room was palpable and I recognised a midwife from Joshua's case. I felt extremely tense and anxious. People were standing up and talking about the fantastic care they had received at FGH Maternity Unit, others paid tribute to the midwives at the Unit and condemned the negative publicity caused by only a small minority of cases.

I summoned the courage to raise my hand to speak. After a few minutes I was given the opportunity. I introduced myself as 'James Titcombe, father of Joshua Titcombe who died due to serious failures in his care at Furness General Hospital in 2008'.

There were loud murmurs and tuts when I spoke, but I carried on. I explained that Joshua had died due to serious failures in his care and that, although such failures only affected a minority, too many other people have lost loved ones in similar ways.

I finished by saying that we would continue to campaign for an inquiry because we wanted the Maternity Unit at FGH to be a safe one. I felt just as strongly as others in the room that Barrow needed a full, consultant-led Maternity Unit at FGH and that I fully supported John Woodcock's campaign to ensure that this was retained.

To my relief, my words were met with applause. John Woodcock gave me strong support at this meeting, and has continued to do so since.

The next week I heard some good news. John Woodcock had secured a meeting with Dan Poulter, now the Under-Secretary of State for Health, to discuss the calls for an inquiry. John invited me to attend and I agreed.

The meeting took place in London on February 12th, 2013. It was a breakthrough moment.

Dan Poulter accepted the need for a fully independent investigation and made a firm commitment that this would happen. The involvement of John Woodcock had been crucial, as well as the support of the other families, especially Liza, Simon and Carl.

The last five years of my life had been totally consumed with Joshua and the repercussions of the events that took place in the 24 hours after his birth. I had been on a journey that had, at times, been almost too much to bear. The sort of very hostile messages I'd seen on the local paper's web pages were something I would have to get used to.

In the months ahead the outcome of some of the processes already triggered would become clear. The external investigation into the CQC's actions at Morecambe Bay was to make international headlines. The Ombudsman eventually investigated my complaint about the NWSHA and the supervisory investigation following Joshua's death, in addition to the complaints made by Carl and Liza. This was to lead to fundamental changes in the regulation of midwifery.

With help from others, we had finally managed to achieve what only a few months ago had seemed impossible. We had a commitment from the government to ensure that a full investigation into the tragic events at Furness General Hospital, including the loss of my much loved and badly missed baby boy, would finally take place.

But the fight was far from over.

Chapter 16 – 'The fish rots from the head'

It is one thing when you find out that your local hospital has suffered serious failures of care resulting in numerous preventable deaths, it is another when you find that hospital is involved, if not in blatant cover-up, in obscuring the extent of the problems. But when you find the organisations responsible for regulating hospitals have not only failed to maintain standards but are complicit in their own cover-ups then you can begin to despair whether you will ever get to the bottom of just how and why these tragedies occurred. This was the picture that began to emerge in 2013.

Things were moving forward, but slowly. Despite the huge sense of relief in knowing that there was now government commitment to a fully independent investigation into Furness General Hospital, the details of when it would actually take place and the specific nature of the investigation remained uncertain.

Dan Poulter had told us that the investigation would still be a locally commissioned process, instigated via the local Clinical Commissioning Group. Would such an investigation be able to look at the full breadth of issues including the role of the regulator and the Ombudsman? The government's view was that no investigation could take place until the criminal investigation had finished. How long would this take?

I discussed these issues with Peter Walsh and DCI Marshall and I didn't see any reason why an independent inquiry couldn't run alongside the police investigation, as long as clear lines of communication were in place.

The information on the Morecambe Bay Inquiry Action website had been attracting a lot of attention; presenting evidence of the scale of problems at FGH in a clear and organised way was a powerful tool. I had been contacted by the Health Editor at the *Sunday Times* who had become very interested in our campaign. On Sunday March 10th, 2013 the *Sunday Times* ran two detailed articles. The story made the front page.

The coverage was well written and convincing. The issues that I'd been working so hard to draw attention to over the last few years now had a national platform.

The article highlighted all the key concerns and issues including the serious questions about the CQC's actions at the Trust. It reported that the CQC had commissioned Grant Thornton, one of the largest consultancy companies in the world, to undertake the investigation and included the following quote from Peter Walsh:

The Morecambe Bay NHS Foundation Trust scandal has almost all the hallmarks of the scandal at Mid Staffs even if not on the same scale... A trust which put its determination to achieve foundation trust status before patient safety, a lack of openness and a failure [by] all the commissioning and regulatory bodies to act quickly to protect patients. The worrying thing is that this all

173

happened after Mid Staffordshire, under a new system. It was
clearly wrong of the CQC to do nothing.

Just two days later on March 12th Dan Poulter announced
that the Department of Health had appointed Dr Bill Kirkup
to chair the independent inquiry into the Trust. Dr Kirkup
had previously been a panel member on the Hillsborough
Independent Investigation. Carl, Liza and I all welcomed
this development.

On March 14th BBC Radio 4's *Today* programme ran
a detailed piece about the problems at Morecambe Bay,
including an interview with myself.

On March 18th I travelled to Manchester to meet the lead
investigator from the Grant Thornton team. I wanted to
ensure that the concerns I had about CQC's actions at the
Trust were properly understood and that all my documentary evidence had been passed over to them. The meeting
was awkward. Absolutely nothing was being given away, but
I was left with a distinct feeling that whatever the investigation had found, it was serious.

I was now in regular email correspondence with the new
Chief Executive at the CQC, David Behan, who had
indicated that the investigation report would be finished
and effectively published by being taken to the CQC Board
meeting on April 25th.

On March 27th the *Telegraph* ran a major article featuring
an interview with Kay Sheldon headlined 'NHS watchdog
approved failing hospitals'.

Kay was very critical of the CQC's actions at Morecambe
Bay, noting that they were 'aware of serious problems by late
2009 and in early 2010, yet in April 2010 the organisation
was registered as fully compliant'.

It just doesn't make sense... There is no way that the Trust could have turned itself round in two or three months. It seems to me that CQC gave assurance about the Trust that wasn't actually accurate... It was a very shocking thing to find, thinking that an organisation that's there to protect patients, had effectively given what amounted to false assurance and that meant that problems in the Trust carried on unacknowledged and unaddressed.

Kay's comments resonated with me. Following Joshua's death I had done everything I could to ensure lessons were learned so that other families wouldn't have to go through what we had suffered. Despite this, we now knew that serious risks to mothers and babies had continued for years. Now a CQC board member was publicly accusing the organisation of giving 'false assurance'. The NHS was not short of organisations which could have done something: the Strategic Health Authority, the Nursing and Midwifery Council, the Health Service Ombudsman, Monitor, the Care Quality Commission - yet no one had taken any action to protect mothers and babies from the very risks that led to Joshua's death.

In the *Telegraph* article Kay said:

CQC had become aware of serious problems at a number of hospitals after those at Mid Staffs had been exposed in 2009, yet did not alert the public because, 'it had been said by the Department of Health that Mid Staffs was a one-off and there was a real sense that finding another Mid Staffs had to be avoided at all costs'.

This suggested that 'not finding another Mid Staffs' was more important than preventing another Mid Staffs from taking place.

Joshua died in November 2008. The final decision by the Ombudsman not to investigate was in February 2010 and the CQC registered the Morecambe Bay Trust 'without conditions' two months later in April - just a month before the May 2010 General Election. Could the failure of the system to highlight and address the scale of problems at Morecambe Bay earlier have been linked to a political desire to avoid bad news about the NHS?

The media interest continued over the next few months. Hardly a week went by without an article about Morecambe Bay and the CQC appearing in the national press. I desperately wanted the truth about what happened at Morecambe Bay to be established; the more media attention there was, the more chance this would happen.

On April 5th Cumbria Police issued the following statement to the press:

Cumbria Constabulary detectives involved in the ongoing police investigation into a number of deaths of mothers and babies that occurred after they received care at Furness General Hospital's maternity unit are now liaising with the independent inquiry team with a view to meeting them, including the independent chair, Dr Bill Kirkup, to share appropriate information.

This course of action is being taken to ensure that clear lines of communication are established so that both the police and independent inquiries can continue side by side without impinging on each other.

I was sure that this announcement had been made after discussing my concerns about the delay with DCI Marshall. I now hoped that this would mean that the Dr Kirkup's investigation could start immediately.

The press attention continued. On April 14th the *Sunday Times* ran an article under the headline 'Father reveals 'cover-up' over his son's death'.

It included the memo to Ann Abraham from her deputy, sent in September 2009 relating to whether or not the Ombudsman would investigate Joshua's case.

In your [Abraham's] conversation with Cynthia Bower [then chief executive of the Care Quality Commission] shortly before our leave, the suggestion arose that if we could assure Mr and Mrs Titcombe that as a result of their experiences CQC are now taking robust action to ensure improvements in the quality of maternity services in the Trust, you might decide not to investigate.

The article also included my recording of the conversation I had with Amanda Sherlock, CQC's director of operations back in September last year.

Sherlock told Titcombe: 'If the Ombudsman had decided to do an investigation into Joshua [in 2010], that would have triggered concerns that we would have looked at as to the organisation's capacity and capability.'

Titcombe sought clarification of her comment.

> *'So the Ombudsman decision not to investigate was like a confidence boost that things were OK?'*

> *'Yes,' replied Sherlock.*

The recording of my conversation with Amanda Sherlock was embedded in the *Sunday Times* article on line so readers could listen to the actual conversation.

The CQC had major questions to answer.

My local MP, John Woodcock, continued to provide strong support and was trying to clarify the status of the investigation. On April 17th John forwarded me a letter from Dan Poulter. The letter was unhelpful to say the least. It stated that the Department of Health was not 'directing the inquiry' and that the process was being directed by the local NHS, who had appointed Dr Kirkup as Chair. On the police investigation, the letter went on to say:

It is our understanding that the police are investigating potentially very serious crimes and this must be allowed to take precedence. However, once a decision is made on whether or not a prosecution will be brought, the situation can be reassessed to see if the independent investigation can get underway.

This appeared to conflict with the announcement from Cumbria Police several days earlier which stated the inquiries could continue 'side by side'.

The CQC had said that the Grant Thornton report would be published on April 25th, just over a week away. I sent David Behan an email asking when the report would be shared with me. On April 19th he replied to say that the CQC would no longer be able to publish the report on the 25th. I emailed David to say I was bitterly disappointed by this news. He apologised and, in his reply, revealed that he believed the CQC got its regulation of Morecambe Bay wrong: 'It is my view that CQC should not have registered Morecambe Bay without conditions'.

The next day the *Health Service Journal* published an 'exclusive' article which stated that David Behan, the new Chief Executive of the CQC, was 'replacing his entire executive director team, including the hiring of a Director of Change'.

It was hard not to draw the conclusion that these announcements were related to the Grant Thornton investigation. This was something the press were soon to pick up on. On May 2nd the *Telegraph* published an article with the headline 'Health Watchdog Sacks Senior Managers Amid Baby Deaths Scandal'.

I continued to push David Behan to confirm when the Grant Thornton report would be published. I was assured that the report would be published in full and shared with me prior to publication, but he could not provide a firm date.

Throughout this time I was in regular contact with Cumbria Police. The police investigation was at a critical stage: DCI Marshall was having meetings with the Crown Prosecution Service to see if the CPS would support a prosecution in relation to Joshua's death. The matter hinged on what is known as 'causation': in the civil litigation system, a successful case can be made if it can be proved that both the standard of care fell below what could have been reasonably expected and that the poor outcome, in the balance of probability, would not have happened were this not the case.

In criminal law, however, the bar for prosecution is not 'in the balance of probability', but 'beyond reasonable doubt'. In Joshua's case there was no doubt that the standard of his care fell significantly below what could have been expected, but the issue of whether Joshua would have survived had he received antibiotics at an appropriate time was now crucial. During Joshua's inquest the Coroner was clear that, in the balance of probability, Joshua would have survived had he received appropriate care. However, we had two different estimates of his chances of survival had he been treated appropriately. The Trust's own expert had stated that this would have been around 90% and, during the inquest, Dr Jane Cassidy, the consultant who cared for Joshua in Newcastle, estimated his chances of survival to be around 80%. I discussed this in depth with DCI Marshall.

I did as much research as I could and even found cases where babies who had the same infection as Joshua but had received antibiotics and had survived. Having lived through the 9 days of Joshua's life, I knew how hard he had fought and how close he came to pulling through. It seemed perverse to me that whether or not the full facts would be allowed to be put before a judge hinged on a technical notion of 'beyond reasonable doubt'. Cumbria Police were doing everything they could to explore this issue, including the commissioning of expert medical reports.

On June 3rd John Woodcock issued a statement expressing his concern over the delay of the publication of the Grant Thornton report.

This report is now months overdue, and those who were tragically affected by the regulatory failures have every right to expect a timely publication of its findings.

On June 6th I finally heard from David Behan. He confirmed that the report would be published via a CQC board meeting on June 19th and that he would travel to meet me in Lancaster two days before to go through the report's findings. David agreed that John Woodcock could attend this meeting.

On Monday June 17th I drove to Lancaster with John Woodcock. The meeting was in a hotel not far from the M6 motorway. When we entered the room I could tell from the look on David Behan's face that we were about to have a very serious meeting. David explained that he was going to go through the key findings with us and that he would give both John and I full copies of the report to take away.

Before going through the report, David stated that it was clear that the CQC had badly failed its regulation of Morecambe Bay and he offered an unreserved apology. He then started to take us through the report. It was more critical than I could have imagined. The key points included:

- An apparent lack of clear procedures, guidelines and effective training for the CQC concerning the registration process

- A general lack of resources, capacity and time to conduct pre-registration inspections

- An over-reliance on Morecambe Bay's self-assessment as part of the application process

- A lack of continuity of oversight by the regional team including the failure by an outgoing manager to pass on key information

- A lack of transparency around how decisions were made

- A less than harmonious and probably dysfunctional working relationship between the Board and the Executive

- A dysfunctional relationship between various stakeholders, including the SHA and CQC. 'We note that these observations echo problems encountered during an earlier period at Mid Staffordshire Foundation Trust'

These were serious issues, but what David Behan said next was truly shocking. He told us that the report concluded that an internal CQC report identifying many of the failures recognised by Grant Thornton may have been deliberately 'covered up'.

When David said these words, John and I looked at each other. Our jaws dropped. I had to stop and ask David - does the report actually use the words 'cover-up'? He referred us to page 15, paragraph 1.50 of the report:

We have carefully considered whether evidence exists to corroborate the assertion that there was an instruction to delete this report. We conclude that such corroborative evidence exists in the form of a contemporaneous note of the meeting and the lack of action taken on the information included in the report... We were also surprised that the fact that such a review took place and was not shared with us during briefings we held with the senior member of management who allegedly gave the instruction to delete the report, ahead of the commencement of our work. We have given careful consideration to whether the alleged instruction to delete the report could in effect constitute a deliberate 'cover-up' and if so what would be the reason for doing so? We have concluded on the balance of the evidence...it might well have constituted a deliberate 'cover-up'.

The report also responded to the specific concerns I had raised about the meeting between the former Chief Executive of the CQC, Cynthia Bower, and the former Health Service Ombudsman, Ann Abraham, before the decision was made by the Ombudsman not to investigate my complaint. The report had concluded that there was nothing improper about the contact between the two organisations but was heavily critical of the CQC for its following actions. The report dismissed my suggestion that these events could have been influenced by external pressure, especially in the light of the May 2010 general election - this was about 'cock-up' not 'conspiracy'. I was not convinced by the reasons given but those issues could wait.

What the report had found was truly shocking. It revealed just how badly the CQC had failed in its regulation of Morecambe Bay and had found evidence of a possible deliberate cover-up of an internal report that had identified these failings.

Families had lost babies due to failures in care at Furness General after 2010, when the CQC had registered the Trust without conditions. The Grant Thornton report had categorically exposed the CQC, the national regulator of the NHS, as being not fit for purpose.

Over the next week there was intense media activity with the story running as a daily headline in most national papers. I was struck by how frank the CQC Chief Executive and Chair were being during this period. When asked about what went wrong within the CQC, David Prior said 'the fish rots from the head'.

It was difficult to think of a more damning expression to describe the CQC's former leadership. This comment didn't come from myself or the other families affected by the failures at Morecambe Bay, but from the CQC itself.

There was no attempt to play down what the Grant Thornton report had revealed and, instead, the emphasis was on the changes that the CQC needed to make to its strategy and culture.

On 20th June, my local MP John Woodcock wrote a column piece that was published in the local paper. I was very touched by what he wrote.

It causes any parent pain even to consider what it would be like to lose a child, so it is genuinely hard to imagine the suffering endured by the Titcombes and other families who lost babies at Furness General Hospital in recent years.

Even worse – if that is possible – if you are convinced your loved ones have been failed, when your battle for basic justice and accountability meets the brick wall of an impenetrable bureaucracy. You get words of sympathy but every attempt to get to the truth is denied or passed to someone else.

It has been a long and often lonely struggle for James Titcombe and other parents who were failed by local health managers and the health watchdog itself, as we now learn.

There were senior officials who created a culture of covering their own backs ahead of ensuring lessons could be learnt and more tragedies.

That is hard to forgive and must never, ever be allowed to return.

When I first met James I thought privately he was a grieving father who had undoubtedly been wronged but who was, probably, seeing conspiracies that did not exist. I was wrong, he was right, and it is only because of his extraordinary tenacity over many years that he has been able to show this appalling wrongdoing to the world with the independent report that has shocked the country this week. Even now, I know there are a minority who suspect the families demanding a public inquiry simply want to damage the hospital.

I just don't think that is right; we can only have confidence in the services we need for future generations if we understand and account for what went wrong in the past. We owe that to patients, but also to nurses and frontline professionals who have also been through an awful time at the hands of weak leaders.

Although I felt very let down by John's early lack of support, I thought these were sincere and courageous words. John continued to provide strong support to myself and other families.

A couple of weeks after the report was released the CQC announced that Kay Sheldon, the CQC board member who had played such an important role in raising the concerns that led to the commissioning of the Grant Thornton report, had been reappointed for a further term. This was a significant step and it gave me real confidence that the CQC was genuinely committed to learn and change.

On June 25th David Behan and David Prior, the CQC Chair, travelled to Barrow to meet the families affected by events at FGH. I had helped organise the meeting and contacted the other families via our Facebook group.

Seven families turned up. David Prior and David Behan talked openly about what the Grant Thornton report had found and offered their unreserved apologies. Each family was then given an opportunity to talk about their experience. It was incredibly moving. Many tears were shed and clear themes emerged from their experiences: midwives had failed or refused to involve doctors when medical help was needed and all but one family said that their experiences of poor care had occurred over a weekend. One of the families explained that they had lost a baby girl on Christmas Day 2010. This was after the CQC had registered the Trust without conditions. Although it was a deeply sad meeting, everyone who attended had a genuine sense that they had been listened to and that the CQC were committed to doing everything possible to learn from what had happened.

I stayed behind after the meeting and had a long conversation with David Prior and David Behan. I talked about the long journey I had been on since losing Joshua, and contrasted the way the NHS systems had responded to Joshua's death with my experience of the safety culture in the nuclear industry. The NHS I had experienced seemed to operate in a culture of fear, where suppressing bad news and covering up mistakes was routine. The experience of my professional life was completely different. I talked about the scheme we currently operated on the project I worked on which incentivised the reporting of safety concerns. Provided that more than 100 'safety observations' were submitted each month to the safety team, one would be pulled from a hat and the winner given an iPad. I talked about how even minor quality issues were investigated to ensure the causes of the issue were identified and any necessary action taken to prevent a recurrence. I also described how we approached individuals who made mistakes. I gave a recent example of someone who was carrying a scaffold pole which he had dropped onto some pipe work below the gantry he was walking on, causing damage to the insulation. The person reported what had happened and was rewarded with a £25 voucher.

Isn't this the culture we should have in the NHS and within the CQC itself?

I stayed in close contact with David Behan and David Prior after this meeting and continued to have a regular dialogue about safety culture and the changes the CQC were making. Over the next few weeks David Behan and I talked about the possibility of my working with the CQC for a 6-month period to help develop their new safety strategy.

Working for an organisation I had been struggling against for many years would be a big step to take. I thought about it a great deal and discussed it at length with Hoa. In the years since Joshua had died I had learned so much about the NHS. I felt I understood some of the gaps and had a clear view on how things could change for the better. It was a difficult decision to leave the company I had worked for over the past 12 years but, in August 2013, I handed in my notice to start working with the CQC from September as their National Advisor on Safety.[5]

In the following weeks I made contact with Bill Kirkup. We met with him in Barrow, along with other families, to agree the terms of reference for the independent investigation. We finally received confirmation that the investigation could proceed in parallel with the police investigation. In addition, the Department of Health confirmed that the investigation would come under its remit rather than being a locally commissioned process. This was all welcome news.

On August 6th I attended a meeting with the Secretary of State for Health, Jeremy Hunt, at Richmond House in Whitehall. I found Jeremy to be warm and caring. I told Joshua's story and he listened intently with tears in his eyes. After discussing patient safety and my experience in the nuclear industry I handed over a document I had written with eight suggestions for making the NHS safer. I have stayed in regular contact with Jeremy Hunt since this first meeting.

This was a significant turning point in my journey. I had spent so much time fighting against the system over the previous five years but now, finally, there seemed to be a genuine acceptance that things were wrong and needed to change. Moreover, I now had an opportunity to influence change from the inside and at a national level.

---

[5] My contract with the CQC was initially for a six-month period. The role of National Advisor on Safety was a new one for the organisation and the first time someone with both a patient background and experience from another safety critical sector had been appointed in an advisory role. At the end of the six-month period, the new role was advertised nationally and I applied. After going through a full interview process I was subsequently offered a permanent job which I decided to accept.

Despite all this positivity, the fight to get to the full truth about the circumstances around Joshua's death and what allowed those conditions to continue was far from over.

On October 5th *Private Eye* published a column which perfectly reflected how complex the circumstances had become.

The Coroner was eventually pursued to open an inquest which was held in 2011 and exposed a cover-up at the Trust. Monitor eventually investigated the Trust in 2011. The CQC eventually investigated the Trust in 2012. Grant Thornton was commissioned to investigate the CQC in 2013 and delivered a scathing verdict of another cover-up. The Ombudsman is currently formally investigating the LSA and the Trust. The Police are formally investigating the Trust. The DoH have commissioned an independent inquiry led by Bill Kirkup to investigate the Trust, the LSA, the CQC and the Ombudsman. Still James waits to find out how and why his son died.

In the months ahead, these processes would eventually take their course, with significant implications not just locally, but for midwifery and for the NHS as a whole.

Chapter 17 – Yet more reports and a change in career

The next few months marked a significant change for me, both personally and professionally. Although there remained many unanswered questions around Joshua's death and the failures at Morecambe Bay, knowing that there was going to be a full independent investigation chaired by Dr Kirkup took a huge weight off my mind. I now needed to let the ongoing processes take their course.

I had a new job and I threw myself into work. This was an exciting time. I was meeting new people in the Patient Safety community, people like me who were dissatisfied by the status quo and passionate about change. I met Martin Bromiley, a truly inspirational man whose wife Elaine died during what should have been a 'routine operation'.

As an airline pilot, Martin recognised that the errors that had led to Elaine's death could be explained by 'Human Factors' - the scientific discipline that is interested in understanding the effects of teamwork, equipment, culture and organisation on human behaviour and performance. This approach was a normal part of his daily life in the airline industry, as it had been in the nuclear industry where I had previously worked.

Martin was amazed to find that in healthcare the under-standing of this discipline was non-existent. He had also expected that an independent investigation into his wife's death would be conducted as a matter of routine for the purposes of learning. He was surprised to find that this was not the case. Martin subsequently set up the Clinical Human Factors Group (CHFG), an independent charity whose work I became involved in. The CHFG has campaigned for almost ten years now and has three main aims. The first is to train and educate health professionals in the science of human factors, the second is to help build organisational systems and cultures that cope well and learn when things go wrong, and the third to develop mechanisms in healthcare for much higher quality investigation and more intelligent approaches to regulation.

I had also come to know Dr Kim Holt, the paediatrician who had blown the whistle on poor care at the clinic in Haringey which subsequently failed to spot injuries sustained by baby Peter Connelly prior to his tragic death (the 'Baby P' case). Kim was co-founder of Patients First, a network of NHS whistleblowers who were campaigning for greater transparency and openness about patient safety issues, and for the NHS to be more open and accountable.

In these two networks I saw great passion and determination combined with practical solutions. Most importantly, I saw clinical staff, managers, patients and carers working together to campaign for badly needed improvements in culture and practice.

On December 10th, 2013 the Parliamentary and Health Service Ombudsman published their report into my complaint about how the Local Supervising Authority and the Strategic Health Authority investigated and responded to

Joshua's death. The report was published together with the complaints made by Carl and Liza and an overarching report titled *Midwifery Supervision and Regulation: recommendation for change.*

The latter report concluded:

We are publishing this report following the completion of three investigations into complaints from three families, all of which related to local midwifery supervision and regulation.

In all three cases, the midwifery supervision and regulatory arrangements at the local level failed to identify poor midwifery practice at Morecambe Bay NHS Foundation Trust. We think these cases clearly illuminate a potential muddling of the supervisory and regulatory roles of Supervisors of Midwives. We think this means that the current system operates in a way that risks failure to learn from mistakes. This cannot be in the interests of the safety of mothers and babies, and must change.

The report made two key recommendations:

- That midwifery supervision and regulation should be separated

- That the NMC should be in direct control of regulatory activity

The report received a lot of media attention, but the response from the midwifery profession was defensive.

Cathy Warwick, Chief Executive of the Royal College of Midwives, was quoted in an article in the *Nursing Times*:

In many maternity services, the supervision of midwives can and should make a significant contribution to the protection of women and their babies... It is very important that the long-term consequences for high-quality maternity care of further changes are very carefully considered. We must be extremely careful not to lose sight of the benefits of midwifery supervision; we could be in danger of throwing the baby out with the bath water.

'Throwing the baby out with the bath water' was an extraordinary choice of phrase in the circumstances but, of more concern - why was the RCM being so defensive about the need for change? Here was a report that found, in three cases, the supervisory system had failed to identify or address clear failures in care that contributed to the deaths of three babies and a mother. Wasn't it obvious that any system of regulation that relied on investigations being carried out by close peers of those involved posed a serious conflict of interest?

The PHSO report was also strongly critical of the North West Strategic Health Authority regarding the way it responded to the complaints Carl, Liza and I made about the LSA investigations in relation to our cases. The former Chief Executive of the NWSHA, Mike Farrar, was now the Chief Executive of the NHS Confederation, the NHS employers' organisation. Just weeks before the PHSO published their report Farrar announced his resignation.

In an article in the *Telegraph* about the PHSO's findings, Farrar was quoted saying 'I remain deeply saddened about the original failings in care at Morecambe Bay Hospital and I apologise unreservedly for the fact that the Strategic Health Authority team was unable to deal with the complaints in the manner families deserved'.

Following the publication of the PHSO report, the NMC commissioned the King's Fund, an influential health policy think tank, to carry out a full review of the recommendations. The King's Fund report supported the recommendations and this led eventually to a commitment from the NMC to change the national framework of midwifery supervision.

The day after the Ombudsman report was published I met with Bill Kirkup and some of the investigation panel members in Preston. I talked through my experience of losing Joshua and what had happened since. It was a difficult thing to do but I wanted to tell Joshua's story in my own words. The panel asked a lot of questions and I left the meeting with a genuine sense that the investigation was going to be robust.

Christmas was always an especially hard time of year. This would be the sixth Christmas since losing Joshua. Emily was now eight years old and Jessica was four. Joshua would have been five. The life I had before Joshua died and the life I was living now were completely different. Joshua had changed everything.

People say that time is a great healer, but I would often still find myself thinking about Joshua and breaking down. While I took huge comfort from the love and happiness of Emily and Jessica, there were always moments when I could not help but think about Joshua. I imagined his excitement as we put up the Christmas decorations and put presents under the tree. Even though it was more than five years since his death, the events at Furness General and those last horrific days in Newcastle were as vivid as ever.

For the past few years I always seemed to be waiting for an investigation or report that would be a milestone, a chance to move forward. First there was the Trust's investigation, then the LSA report and various subsequent appeals and complaints, then our complaint to the Ombudsman, then the inquest, then the investigation into CQC's actions at Morecambe Bay. We were still waiting for the outcome of the police investigation and Bill Kirkup's independent investigation but we knew these would take some time.

The next milestone would be the publication of four further reports from the Ombudsman. The first report was about how the Trust handled my complaints into the events around Joshua's death, the second and third about offensive or inappropriate email correspondences (the 'NMC shit' and 'Has JT has moved to Thailand' emails) and the fourth about the way the Trust had prepared answers prior to Joshua's inquest.

On February 27th the Ombudsman's reports were finally published. They fully upheld my complaint about the way the Trust responded to Joshua's death and the email correspondence we had uncovered.

The foreword stated:

The investigations in this report follow the avoidable death of a baby. Our investigations are about a father's attempts to find out what happened and his desire to improve patient safety, to prevent the same thing happening to others.

The Trust could only achieve these things if they answered the family's questions openly and honestly and learnt from what they found.

We have concluded that the Trust did not do this. This is particularly unacceptable when an avoidable death was the cause of the complaints. The fact that the early records were missing compounded the problem. Looking at all of the complaints together, they demonstrate that a lack of openness by the Trust and the quality of their investigations of these complaints caused a loss of trust and further pain for the family.

The report made some strong recommendations for change:

Cultural change is needed from the ward to the board. Openness and learning must be strongly led and must start with definitive action by hospital boards. Hospital boards should establish expectations of openness and honesty, seeking feedback in order to learn and improve. They should reward staff who seek and respond well to concerns and complaints, including acknowledging mistakes. This will foster a new culture of remedy and learning.

Some recommendations on how investigations of healthcare failures should be carried out were also made:

Looking at the root cause of the problem that leads to a complaint and the interactions between people involved are critical tools in helping to learn from complaints. The science of Human Factors seeks to understand the effects of teamwork, tasks, equipment, workspace, culture and organisation on human behaviour. We will expect these tools to be used in future independent investigations.

My family and I welcomed these recommendations, but I did wonder how they were going to be followed through and implemented. I was aware, from both the many other families with tragic stories that I knew personally and through people I had met through my role at the CQC, that poor quality investigations and the way organisations responded to avoidable harm were major national issues. If there was any single thing that I wanted Joshua's story to change, it was how the NHS responded to and learned from mistakes. Despite my previous awful experiences with the PHSO, I was grateful that their report had made these recommendations which I hoped would add to the momentum of the patient safety movement and lead to change.

However, the fourth report into the Trust and the possible collusion with the midwives prior to the inquest was deeply disappointing. The Ombudsman had completely rejected my complaint, stating that their investigation had found the inquest preparations were in accordance with 'good practice', and that there was no evidence that midwives had colluded regarding the evidence they gave at the inquest. The Ombudsman accepted they were all ignorant that Joshua's low temperature could have been a sign of neonatal sepsis. We simply couldn't believe that the Ombudsman had reached this conclusion - the evidence seemed so clear. The Coroner himself during his summing up suggested there had been collaboration. Following this, I had managed to obtain an actual document that appeared to show possible questions and model answers relating to Joshua's care that had been distributed to Trust witnesses prior to the inquest.

The Ombudsman had refused to investigate Joshua's case after my initial referral in 2009, yet when they did eventually look at how the Trust responded to Joshua's death years later, they found serious failures and 'maladministration'. The Ombudsman had also refused to investigate my complaint about the supervisory investigation into Joshua's death, yet following the start of a Judicial Review process and complaints made by other families, they eventually investigated only to find serious failures which led to recommendations for national changes. The Ombudsman's report into my complaint about collusion was long and extremely detailed, but I felt strongly that none of the explanations or logic behind the decision stood up to scrutiny.

My family and I made it clear that we completely rejected this fourth report. I was confident that the independent investigation chaired by Bill Kirkup would re-examine these issues and reach a more satisfactory conclusion.

The Ombudsman's reports featured in both the national and local press. It soon became clear that some did not welcome any more interest in the failures at Furness General Hospital. On March 18th a friend drew my attention to a letter published in the local paper. It was from a Dr Rowlatt and read:

YET again you give space to James Titcombe following the tragic and avoidable death of his newborn baby son Joshua in November 2008.

Is it not time for Mr Titcombe to let Joshua's soul rest in peace?

Mr Titcombe is not the only one whose life has been made hell by this affair. It does not seem to worry him that his activities may have caused more harm than good to the maternity unit at Furness General. Far from exposing the truth, he may have obscured it.

He must have cost the NHS many thousands of pounds in lawsuits, in enquiries and in the dismissal of senior midwives. Only malpractice lawyers can gain any satisfaction from this.

What if Mr Titcombe disagrees with Dr Kirkup's report into the maternity services of Morecambe Bay Hospitals?

I was deeply upset by this letter. I had been on such a long and difficult journey since losing Joshua. At first we had faced so much denial that the problems at FGH were wider than Joshua's loss alone, but by now there had been so many reports that showed how serious the problems were that there could be little doubt that the failures in care continued for years after Joshua had died.

None of this would have come to light were it not for the hard campaigning and fighting by myself and the other families. However uncomfortable it was for local people to read about the problems, wasn't it much better for the truth to be heard and the problems faced up to, rather than serious issues being swept under the carpet?

What did this man know about how hard I had tried to 'let Joshua's soul rest in peace'? How could any father do this when there had been so much dishonesty and cover-up? Nothing I did over the last six years had felt like a choice – rather, it had been an excruciatingly painful and unwanted battle that I had no option but to be part of.

How could anyone, let alone a doctor, argue that the only people to gain from my efforts to highlight the truth were 'malpractice lawyers'?

It seems that whenever a tragedy in healthcare like the preventable death of a baby occurs, many want to forget the painful truth and 'move on', arguing that however lamentable the event, nothing will bring the child back. Continuing to go over the case will only cause the professionals involved further stress and mistrust, holding back the service from growing.

This might be an understandable human reaction but it not only undervalues the pain felt by those who have directly suffered the loss but, crucially, it prevents organisations from learning just how these mistakes happened and how we can stop them happening again.

The rest of 2014 went by quickly. I was enjoying my new role working with the CQC. I found myself among a small but growing network of people dedicated to patient safety.

It was originally anticipated that the Kirkup investigation would be completed by the end of the summer. When it failed to appear I was hopeful the report could still be completed before the end of the year but, as Christmas of 2014 approached, it became clear that this wasn't going to happen.

After Christmas I heard the final report would be published

toward the end of February 2015 - most likely the week of Monday 23rd. I had a long discussion about the publication with Hoa; we expected that there would be some media attention around the report and it would be a good idea if Hoa took the girls to visit her parents in Vietnam. She arranged to fly out to Hanoi on February 12th and to return on March 4th.

On February 13th, the day after Hoa and the girls had left, the publication date was delayed yet again until the week of March 2nd. This was really disappointing, not least because it meant Hoa and the girls might be back at home when the report was published, something we had hoped to avoid.

With the announcement of this delay, I decided to go to Hanoi to spend a few weeks with Hoa, Emily and Jessica. I flew out on Tuesday February 17th with my return flight booked to land in Manchester in the early hours of the morning on March 2nd. I needed to get away and a trip to Vietnam would be the perfect distraction.

It was a lovely holiday. I arrived in Hanoi just in time for the Vietnamese New Year celebrations on Thursday 19th. I walked with Hoa, Emily and Jessica around Hoan Kiem Lake in the centre of Hanoi and watched the fireworks and celebrations, followed by a traditional family meal with Hoa's parents in the early hours of the morning. I have always loved Vietnam and the sights and sounds of Hanoi reminded me of when I first met Hoa, all those years ago. So much had changed in our lives since then, but Hanoi seemed just as enthralling and exciting as it had always been.

We spent the first week in Hanoi catching up with family and enjoying the city. We then went away to a resort in Ninh Binh province, a two-hour car journey away. While we were in Ninh Binh the investigation team emailed me to say the report would be published on March 3rd at a press conference at the Grange Hotel in Cumbria. Bill Kirkup would be briefing families at a venue in Barrow on the evening of Monday 2nd - the same day as I was due to land back in England.

The rest of the holiday went by quickly. After the trip to Ninh Binh we returned to Hanoi for a few more days. It was soon time for me to leave for the airport. I said goodbye to Hoa and the girls and headed off by taxi. On the flight home, I could think of nothing but the investigation report and what it was going to say. I was not going to have to wait long to find out.

Chapter 18 - The Kirkup Report

To err is human, to cover up is unforgivable, and to fail to learn is inexcusable.

- Sir Liam Donaldson

I landed at Manchester Airport on Monday, March 2nd just after 6am. I caught the first train I could and got back home around midday. I was so tired that I went straight to sleep and slept right through until my alarm went off at 6pm. After a shower it was time to go and meet Bill Kirkup at the venue in Barrow. I arrived a few minutes before the meeting started at 7pm.

Many other families were there, some of whom I had never met before. What happened at FGH had affected so many lives; this was about far more than Joshua and the experience of my family.

The room was quiet. All the families present were nervous about what they were about to hear. Despite everything I had learned over the years, despite how obvious the truth appeared, a small part of me feared this investigation might be another let down, leaving yet more unanswered questions.

Dr Kirkup arrived and we all sat in silence. After a brief introduction we were taken through the findings of the investigation.

Dr Kirkup described the Maternity Unit at FGH as being seriously dysfunctional. Clinical competence was substandard. Staff had deficient skills and knowledge and working relationships were extremely poor, particularly between different staff groups, such as obstetricians, paediatricians and midwives. He described a culture among midwives of pursuing normal childbirth 'at any cost' and his investigation had found widespread failures of risk assessment and care planning resulting in inappropriate and unsafe care. The response to adverse incidents was grossly deficient and there had been repeated failures to investigate properly and learn lessons.

These factors had combined to create what he described as a 'lethal mix', leading to the unnecessary deaths of mothers and babies.

The investigation had reviewed all the maternal deaths and deaths of babies under the period of investigation and had found 20 instances of 'significant or major failures of care' at Furness General. These were associated with the deaths of three mothers and 16 babies, almost four times the number of failures of care at the Royal Lancaster Infirmary, another of the Trust's Maternity Units, which had a higher number of births per year.

Dr Kirkup described a pattern of failure to recognise problems. There were missed opportunities to intervene at almost every level of the NHS. This included the Strategic Health Authority, the Care Quality Commission, the Health Service Ombudsman right up to the Department of Health.

The reaction from Maternity Unit staff had been shaped by denial that there was a problem and a strong rejection of criticism. The report described the supposed universal lack of knowledge of the significance of Joshua's hypothermia as clear evidence of 'distortion of the truth'. Importantly, the investigation had reached a clear finding on how the Trust and staff prepared prior to Joshua's inquest. Despite an Ombudsman's report that rejected my complaint, Dr Kirkup's report was highly critical. The investigation had concluded that this was 'evidence of inappropriate distortion of the process of preparation for an inquest'.

None of the families at the meeting were given a copy of the report - we would have to wait until the press conference the following day at Grange-over-Sands, a 30-minute drive from Barrow. The families who attended the press conference would be given the opportunity to read the report at 10am the following day, two hours before the conference started.

I had heard enough to realise that the review had not pulled any punches. What Dr Kirkup described was consistent with everything I had learned over the last six years. Finally we would have an independent investigation report that would provide the truth that I and so many other families were hoping for.

I left the meeting with a sense of relief, but anxious about the press conference the following day and eager to read the details of the full report.

I slept well that night, still tired from the long flight back from Vietnam. The next day I woke up early and went to Joshua's grave in a cemetery just a short walk from our house. It was a warm, sunny morning and I sat for a while and thought. After all these years, a report was about to be published that finally told the full truth about why my beautiful baby boy had died in the way he had, from a condition that could have easily been treated with the most basic of medical care. I knew that this report was not going to be a source of celebration or happiness; whatever it said, however damning it was about these events, it wasn't going to change the one thing in the world I wanted. It couldn't bring Joshua back. I was quite alone. I closed my eyes and told Joshua how much I loved him and then walked back to the house and set off for Grange-over-Sands.

I arrived just after 10am. I was given a full copy of the report and directed to an area of the hotel where other families were already reading through their copies. There were more faces that I didn't recognise. I sat down and started to read the report in detail.

After reading through all 221 pages, although I fully agreed with the vast majority of the findings and conclusions, there were still a few areas that I struggled to fully accept. The report was a meticulous and thorough investigation of the events at the Trust itself, the clinical failures that occurred and how the local and national system responded. However the report, although highly critical of almost every organisation involved, concluded, just as Grant Thornton had done back in 2013, that the failures of the wider system to highlight and intervene earlier was 'cock-up' rather than 'conspiracy'. To this day I am not convinced that there wasn't at least an element of deliberate suppression through a desire to keep 'bad news' about the NHS quiet, especially in the run up to the 2010 general election. These are complex issues and invariably difficult to prove.[6]

---

[6] See Appendix 2 for my letter to Bill Kirkup, presenting the questions that still remain unanswered.

This issue aside, the vast majority of the report rang true for me and it was a huge vindication of everything I had been fighting to prove for so long.

The introduction read:

These events have finally been brought to light thanks to the efforts of some diligent and courageous families, who persistently refused to accept what they were being told. Those families deserve great credit. That it needed their efforts over such a prolonged period reflects little credit on any of the NHS organisations concerned. Today, the name of Morecambe Bay has been added to a roll of dishonoured NHS names that stretches from Ely Hospital to Mid Staffordshire.

The report's overall conclusion was well summarised in the following paragraphs from the executive summary:

Our conclusion is that these events represent a major failure at almost every level. There were clinical failures, including failures of knowledge, team-working and approach to risk. There were investigatory failures, so that problems were not recognised and the same mistakes were needlessly repeated. There were failures, by both Maternity Unit staff and senior Trust staff, to escalate clear concerns that posed a threat to safety. There were repeated failures to be honest and open with patients, relatives and others raising concerns. The Trust was not honest and open with external bodies or the public. There was significant organisational failure on the part of the CQC, which left it unable to respond effectively to evidence of problems. The NWSHA and the PHSO failed to take opportunities that could have brought the problems to light sooner, and the DH was reliant on misleadingly optimistic assessments from the NWSHA. All of these organisations failed to work together effectively and to communicate effectively, and the result was mutual reassurance concerning the Trust that was based on no substance.

We found at least seven significant missed opportunities to inter-vene over the three years from 2008 (and two previously), across each level – from the FGH Maternity Unit upwards.

Tragically and most distressingly for me, the report con-firmed that deaths continued to happen long after 2008:

Since 2008, there have been ten deaths in which there were significant or major failures of care; different clinical care in six would have been expected to prevent the outcome.

Despite everything I had tried to do to ensure lessons were learned following Joshua's death, at least six more lives were subsequently lost as a result of ongoing failures.

I thought back to the letter I wrote to Ann Abraham (the former Ombudsman) in February 2010 after PHSO had refused to investigate Joshua's death:

I have begged and begged for your help, not because I want compensation, not because I think you can bring Joshua back, but because I genuinely don't want to see any other family go through the experience we have. I believe with all my heart that you have missed an opportunity to ensure that what happened, after Joshua died, is never repeated again.

Dr Kirkup's report confirmed that PHSO had missed opportunities to bring the problems at FGH to light sooner.

The report was also very critical of the CQC's actions at the time:

The organisation that most clearly failed to deal adequately with the Trust was the CQC. It was newly formed in April 2009 from the merger of two large organisations and a smaller one, with a very broad remit for regulation of the whole health and social care sector. It is clear from the example of this Trust that the way it set about these tasks was wholly inadequate, and the results were the series of inconsistent judgments, communication breakdowns and misdirected visits that we have set out.

It did feel strange reading about such serious criticism of an organisation that I now worked for, but I didn't feel at all conflicted. When I made the decision to join the CQC more than a year earlier, it was in the knowledge that I was joining an organisation that fully accepted where it had gone wrong in the past and was committed to change. Since then, I had actually been involved in the changes from the inside. I knew that the CQC were still only part way through their journey, but I had no doubt that things had moved on significantly and were continuing in the right direction.

The report was critical about the Trust's preoccupation with achieving Foundation Trust status:

The Trust was heavily focused on achieving Foundation Trust (FT) status, and this played a significant part in what transpired.

Dr Kirkup's report also discussed the Fielding Report, the highly critical review of maternity services at FGH that had been disclosed to me as part of Joshua's inquest preparations and which was eventually sent to the regulators by me, long after the Trust had been awarded FT status. The Kirkup report concluded:

Although we heard different accounts, and it was clear that there was limited managerial capacity to deal with a demanding agenda, including the FT application, we found on the balance of probability that there was an element of conscious suppression of the report both internally and externally.

This was a damning conclusion. A report which revealed serious concerns about risk to mothers and babies at FGH was likely to have been deliberately suppressed in order to help the Trust achieve its objective of becoming an FT. How could an organisational culture become so twisted that it prioritised achieving a strategic objective above the safety of mothers and babies?

Dr Kirkup's report concluded that the SHA, the organisation responsible for ensuring standards in midwifery supervision, had provided a 'misleading' brief to the Department of Health, stating that its view was that the serious untoward incidents at FGH Maternity Unit in 2008, which included Joshua's death, were 'coincidental'. The report concluded that:

...had the SHA 'adopted a more 'hands-on' approach, it is likely that both the implementation of action plans and the unconnected nature of the incidents would have been challenged. This was another missed opportunity.

The report was not just critical of managers and external regulators and governance organisations, it was also critical of the behaviour and action of individuals:

We make no criticism of staff for individual errors which, for the most part, happen despite their best efforts and are found in all healthcare systems. Where individuals collude in concealing the truth of what has happened, however, their behaviour is inexcusable, as well as unprofessional. The failure to present a complete picture of how the Maternity Unit was operating was a missed opportunity that delayed both recognition and resolution of the problems and put further women and babies at risk.

The report highlighted some particular issues directly related to Joshua's case:

Many of the reactions of Maternity Unit staff at this stage were shaped by denial that there was a problem, their rejection of criticism of them that they felt was unjustified (and which, on occasion, turned to hostility) and a strong group mentality amongst midwives characterised as 'the musketeers'. We found clear evidence of distortion of the truth in responses to investigation, including particularly the supposed universal lack of knowledge of the significance of hypothermia in a newborn baby, and in this context events such as the disappearance of records, although capable of innocent explanation, concerned us. We also found evidence of inappropriate distortion of the process of preparation for an inquest, with circulation of what we could only describe as 'model answers'.

I had always maintained that the evidence the midwives gave during Joshua's inquest, with not one of them knowing Joshua's low temperature was a sign of infection, simply could not have been the truth. After a long investigation, the PHSO had rejected my complaint. Here I was in March 2015, nearly four years after his inquest and more than six years after Joshua died, finally reading the obvious truth:

Any clinically qualified member of staff looking after neonates should be aware that a failure to maintain temperature is a cardinal sign of infection in a neonate, and Joshua was under observation for potential infection following his mother's illness and spontaneous rupture of the membranes. The account subsequently given by every midwife involved, including to the inquest into Joshua's death, was that none of them knew that hypothermia in a neonate could signify infection or should have resulted in an urgent paediatric assessment. It is on the face of it extraordinary that not a single one knew this basic fact, and many experienced interviewees expressed varying degrees of surprise and disbelief (one Local Supervising Authority (LSA) midwife said to us that a unit in which no midwife knew this would have been unique in her experience)... This represents a significant and regrettable attempt to conceal an evident truth, that a cardinal sign of infection in a newborn baby was wrongly ignored.

For the first time, despite going through the entirety of the NHS complaints process, including a PHSO investigation, we now also had the truth about how the Trust prepared for Joshua's inquest.

A meeting took place to prepare the midwives who had been asked to give evidence. This would be entirely in order, and appropriate, given that most would not previously have been involved in such a process, and information on what would happen and what would be expected of them would be helpful both to them and to the process. As part of that meeting, a solicitor working for the Trust's legal advisors presented a series of 'difficult questions' that she felt witnesses were likely to be asked. This would be more controversial, but not in itself improper, provided that there was no general discussion of how to respond, on which both documentary evidence and interviewees are silent. What happened next, however, was clearly wrong: Jeanette Parkinson, the Maternity Risk Manager and Senior Midwife, prepared a single set of what we can only regard as 'model answers' to the questions, and circulated them to all of the midwives involved. This distortion of the process underlying an inquest was picked up by the Coroner, who commented on the similarity of the accounts that he heard from different witnesses and the concern that this caused him.

The report stated that midwifery care in the unit at FGH:

...became strongly influenced by a small number of dominant individuals whose over-zealous pursuit of the natural childbirth approach led at times to inappropriate and unsafe care.

An interviewee said:

There were a group of midwives who thought that normal childbirth was the... be all and end all... at any cost... yeah, it does sound awful, but I think it's true – you have a normal delivery at any cost.

There was a strong view among staff that they were being unfairly criticised which on occasions became overt hostility:

This underlying feeling was evident at times from the approach taken by interviewees in responding to our questions, and was sometimes apparent in email correspondence. The most notable example is an email from one midwife to another concerning a Nursing and Midwifery Council (NMC) investigation that was entitled 'NMC Shit'. There is no excuse for committing such views to the record, but more important is the underlying attitude it illustrates.

The report quoted one midwife saying 'sometimes bad things happen in maternity – people just have to accept it'.

Although I had lived and breathed these issues for the last six years, it was still shocking to see the facts so clearly laid out on paper.

The report made a total of 44 recommendations: 18 for the Morecambe Bay Trust and 26 for the wider NHS. I agreed with all of them but, if I had to choose just one that I felt was needed to drive change more than any other, it would have been recommendation 23:

Clear standards should be drawn up for incident reporting and investigation in maternity services. These should include the mandatory reporting and investigation as serious incidents of maternal deaths, late and intrapartum stillbirths and unexpected neonatal deaths. We believe that there is a strong case to include a requirement that investigation of these incidents be subject to a standardised process, which includes input from and feedback to families, and independent, multidisciplinary peer review, and should certainly be framed to exclude conflicts of interest between staff.

In all that had happened since Joshua's death, the biggest tragedy for me was that even after Joshua died in horrific circumstances, lessons weren't learned to protect other mothers and babies from the very same risks. The Kirkup report confirmed that the failure to learn from events that ought to have triggered change, went back long before Joshua's death.

As I finish the final chapter of Joshua's story, I must go right back to close to where the story started.

On the day of Joshua's funeral I was standing in a flower shop in Dalton, buying some flowers for his grave. The lady asked 'are they for someone special?' and when I explained the circumstances, she broke down into tears, telling me that she had lost a baby at FGH in 2004, but that in her case, it was 'just one of those things'.

The Kirkup report described this very case:

The first event that should have triggered concern was the death shortly after delivery of a normal, term baby...in 2004. However, the investigation that was carried out was rudimentary, protective of the midwife involved, and failed to identify the shortcomings in practice and approach that led to inadequate monitoring of a high-risk pregnancy and a lack of necessary obstetric assessment and intervention...Had an effective multidisciplinary investigation been carried out, it is likely that the early stages of dysfunctional relationships and inappropriate risk assessment would have been identified and could have been addressed, as the case shows several of the features that would become familiar later, including poor assessment of risk and failure to monitor adequately.

If this had been done in 2004, it would not only have reduced the likelihood of unnecessary loss of babies and mothers, it could have corrected the poor risk assessment and unsafe practice at an early stage, before inappropriate attitudes and behaviour had become more deeply embedded into day-to-day practice and influenced others on the Unit.

Of course, I could not read these words without thinking of Joshua. The course of events for my son and so many others would surely have been different if only there had been openness and honesty when this early tragedy occurred.

More than six years after our precious baby son died, with the help of other brave families, the media and some key individuals who, at critical times, went against the prevailing tide to provide support and help, we had finally managed to make sense of the sequence of events that led to Joshua's death and the loss of so many other innocent lives.

It is a story that I dearly wish I had never had the need to write, and one I hope politicians, healthcare leaders and NHS staff will heed and work together to ensure similar events are never allowed to happen again.

Afterword

On April 24th, 2015 Cumbria Police announced that the criminal investigation into Joshua's death had concluded without any prosecutions.

As the Kirkup investigation acknowledged, the bar for criminal prosecution is for the police to prove beyond all reasonable doubt that a crime has been committed, which in this case was always going to be very difficult.

On July 16th the government published its response to the Morecambe Bay Investigation, as part of its *Learning not Blaming* report. The government accepted all the report's recommendations. The report also confirmed a commitment from the government to reform the regulatory system for midwives and to establish an independent patient safety investigation body to be operational by April 2016.

At the time of writing, the Nursing and Midwifery Council (NMC) are still carrying out Fitness to Practice investigations relating to five registrants involved in Joshua's care.

On September 15th, 2015 after a prolonged battle the PHSO agreed to take their report about Joshua's inquest preparations off the PHSO website. In a letter to me from the PHSO, Dame Julie Mellor stated:

We were unable to determine whether an allegation of collusion amongst the midwives in preparation for the inquest occurred and know you remain unhappy with this decision.

We recognise that our decision to publish this information and subsequent correspondence on our website had been particularly upsetting for you and has caused you distress which we could have avoided. I am very sorry for this... We acknowledge that we need to modernise our service and culture... We recognise that in future when considering complaints of collusion, we need to look at whether we are able to gather enough evidence in order to come to sound findings.

Joshua's Story – Timeline of events

2008

July 31st   Nittaya Hendrickson dies at FGH and baby Chester shortly after

September 6th   Baby Alex Brady dies at Furness General Hospital

October 27th   Baby Joshua Titcombe born at FGH

November 5th   Baby Joshua dies at the Freeman Hospital in Newcastle

November 14th   James Titcombe (JT) submits detailed chronology of Joshua's care to United Hospitals Morecambe Bay NHS Trust (UHMB) Chief Executive, Tony Halsall

November 25th   UHMB Customer Service Manager confirms Joshua's observation records have 'gone missing'

December 9th   JT writes to the Coroner in Newcastle but an inquest is refused

2009

February	UHMB internal investigation report into Joshua's death released
April 4th	Initial letter to the Parliamentary and Health Service Ombudsman (PHSO) requesting an investigation into Joshua's death
April 18th	Joshua's death is reported in the *North West Evening Mail*
May	Care Quality Commission (CQC) learns of 12 Serious Untoward Incidents reported by UHMB – five relating to maternity services
June 1st	Local Supervising Authority (LSA) complete report into Joshua's death
July	Titcombe family accepts settlement from NHS Litigation Authority
December	CQC's Regional Director details a number of serious concerns about UHMB and maternity services at FGH

2010

February 3rd	PHSO confirm their decision not to investigate Joshua's death
February 5th	JT writes to the Coroner in Newcastle again to request an inquest
March	UHMB receives the first version of Fielding report

March 19th	Tony Halsall writes that he is 'drawing the complaints process to an end'
March 24th	Newcastle Coroner David Mitford confirms that an inquest into Joshua's death will be opened
June	CQC carries out an unannounced inspection of FGH and gives it a clean bill of health
June 25th	The Northwest Strategic Health Authority (NWSHA) complete their review of the LSA report into Joshua's death concluding it was carried out in accordance with policy
October 1st	Monitor authorises Foundation status to UHMB
November 19th	Meeting with the NWSHA and NMC finally accepts the LSA investigation was flawed

2011

January 7th	'NMC Shit' email revealed
January 21st	JT sends Fielding report to the CQC
February 25th	NWSHA refuses request for a second LSA investigation into Joshua's death
March 9th	Detailed complaint sent to PHSO about the LSA report into Joshua's death and the NWHSA's response

March 30th	Cumbria Police start a formal investigation
June 2nd – 6th	Inquest into Joshua's death in Cumbria
June	Police widen investigation to include other families who had received care at FGH
June 13th	PHSO reject the complaint made about the LSA report and NWSHA response
September	CQC publish a damning inspection report - UHMB fails to meet six essential standards with three major concerns
October	Monitor find UHMB in 'significant breach' of its terms of authorisation
	Dr Foster mortality figures place UHMB as the worst performing in the country

2012

February 7th	Monitor publishes three further critical reports, including one into maternity services identifying 119 'unaddressed risks'
February 24th	UHMB Chief Executive Tony Halsall resigns
March 22nd	JT sends detailed 'letter before claim' to the PHSO to start of Judicial Review proceedings against the decision not to investigate complaint about the LSA/ NWSHA

March 30th	Concerns raised in *Telegraph* re CQC's actions, quoting CQC board member Kay Sheldon
May	PHSO complete second review of decision not to investigate JT's complaint about the LSA/NWSHA. The review states the original decision 'does not stand up to scrutiny' and recommends the complaint is reconsidered
July 15th	*Sunday Post* runs JT's call for a public inquiry on the front page
August	CQC confirms they are reviewing regulatory actions at UHMB
November	JT meets CQC's new Chief Executive David Behan. Terms of reference for the Grant Thornton review are extended to include concerns prior to April 2010
December	Joshua's story aired on BBC1 *Panorama* as part of a programme about safety in hospitals

2013

January	PHSO agrees to investigate UHMB response to Joshua's death, concerns about collusion at the inquest and offensive email correspondence
January 30th	Morecambe Bay Inquiry Action launch campaign in Barrow

February 12th	JT meets Dan Poulter MP and John Woodcock MP. Dan Poulter confirms government support for a fully independent investigation of events at UHMB
March 12th	Dr Bill Kirkup announced as Chair of the Morecambe Bay Investigation
June 19th	Grant Thornton report into CQC's regulator failures at UHMB published. The report makes front page news for more than a week
September	JT starts working for CQC as an Advisor on Safety
December	PHSO publish their investigation into the LSA investigation into Joshua's death and similar complaints by two other families. The report finds maladministration in all three cases and recommends changes to the national system of midwifery regulation

2014

January	NMC commissions the King's Fund to review the PHSO recommendations on the statutory regulation of midwives
February	PHSO publish four reports relating to complaints about Joshua. Three are upheld but the fourth report concludes that Joshua's inquest preparations were 'in line with good practice'

2015

January 28th   NMC Council accept the key recommendation of the King's Fund review into statutory supervision of midwives

March 3rd   Kirkup report published

April   Cumbria Police close criminal investigation into Joshua's death with no prosecutions

July   Government publishes *Learning Not Blaming* report and accepts all the Kirkup report's recommendations

September   PHSO remove their report relating to Joshua's inquest from their website, issuing an apology for the distress caused

Links

Action against Medical Accidents (AvMA)

AvMA is a leading UK charity for patient safety and justice. They provide free independent advice and support to people affected by medical accidents through a specialist helpline, written casework and inquest support services

www.avma.org.uk

Sands - the Stillbirth and neonatal death charity

Sands operates throughout the UK, supporting anyone affected by the death of a baby, working to improve the care bereaved parents receive and promoting research to reduce the loss of babies' lives.

www.uk-sands.org

Patients Association

The Patients Association is a national healthcare charity promoting the voice of patients in health services

www.patients-association.org.uk

The Clinical Human Factors Group (CHFG)

The Clinical Human Factors Group is a broad coalition of healthcare professionals, managers and service-users who have partnered with experts in Human Factors from health-care and other high-risk industries to campaign for change in the NHS.

www.chfg.org

Patient Stories

Patient Stories uses digital and broadcast media approaches to provoke debate about safety and patient experience in healthcare.

Information and resources, including a film about Joshua's Story are available here.

www.patientstories.org.uk

Appendix 1

Alex Davey-Brady's story, prepared by
Alex's Mother and Father

Our beautiful, perfect baby boy died as a result of failings at
Furness General Hospital on September 6th, 2008.

On an early trip to see our consultant we were reassured that we
would be looked after in our second pregnancy. This helped put our
minds at rest after a difficult first labour with our first son Tyler
in 2005. The consultant explained if the baby was to be of a large
size they would consider early induction. It was documented we
were to see the consultant again in the last stage of pregnancy.
After repeated requests from us we never saw our consultant
again.

As the pregnancy steadily progressed so did Alex's estimated
weight. Tyler was born weighing 8lb 6oz and yet at only 32
weeks gone, Alex was already creeping up on this weight. To say
we were concerned would be a huge understatement and when
we questioned his gaining size it was treated with amusement
by the midwives.

At 39 weeks we spoke to a consultant about our concerns; Alex
was now estimated to be around 10lbs and after discussion they

agreed I could be induced and during labour a cannula would be in place in case an emergency caesarean needed to take place. We were finally going to meet our little boy.

After induction started it took nearly 24 hours for things to start moving; labour progressed very slowly and after repeatedly requesting a caesarean, a request which was ignored, a consultant was finally called to examine me. The consultant arrived and never even came to examine me; I was left in the hands of the midwife ignoring my requests.

Shortly after 9pm Alex's heart rate showed he was in distress and the doctor went to get changed for an instrumental delivery; he didn't come back for almost 30 minutes. The midwife was determined to deliver Alex even when the doctor returned – it was clear there was tension between the midwives and doctors. After being put into all positions the doctor had enough of standing back and overruled the midwives and delivered Alex with difficulty due to shoulder dystocia.

Alex was born at 21.39 weighing 11lb 13 1/2ozs on the 6/9/08 – numbers that I'll never forget. All Alex ever had were these three sets of numbers and they will forever be etched on my mind.

Alex was born with the umbilical cord wrapped around his neck and sadly didn't respond to any resuscitation.

The news came that our little boy had died, we were never going to see our little man open his eyes.

A pain we've never experienced took over us that night but instinctively we knew things had gone wrong, preventable things that if a suitable birth plan had been in place or if midwives and consultants had acted sooner I wouldn't be here writing this today and our little boy would be here with us.

I was unable to hold my baby boy as I was too scared I wouldn't be able to let him go. Simon held him for hours, he was perfect and looked just like our eldest son Tyler.

The next morning we picked out some clothes for him to wear; we didn't have many things with us that fit him due to his large size. Leaving the hospital that day without our baby is the hardest thing we have ever had to do and to go home where his room is set up ready was heart breaking. The pain was unbearable.

Within twenty four hours we had contacted the trust's complaints department and expressed our concerns and a date was agreed to make statements.

In the meantime we were contacted by the coroner's office who had been alerted to what had happened and assured us they would be investigating and they would now look after Alex. Having to carry my little boy into the church in his coffin was the hardest and most surreal thing I have ever had to do and to this day still have nightmares of dropping him and destroying what were my final duties for him.

6 weeks after Alex's death a consultant wrote an email to his colleagues expressing he had 'grave concerns' regarding the care I received and stated 'this has happened in our unit in the past and if we don't take appropriate action this will happen again in the future'.

Alex's inquest was 10 months later. The Coroner stated "The midwives ran the show"; it reflected how we felt of the events from that night. He then issued a Rule 43 Letter to see what improvement have been made.

After a three year battle filled with lies, cover ups and many tears shed the trust finally admitted liability for my son's death. They could not possibly defend not monitoring his heartbeat correctly or not having a suitable birth plan in place for a baby weighing nearly twelve pounds. We hoped lessons would be learned at the hospital after Alex's preventable death but have learned similar mistakes had been going on before and after our tragic loss.

When we lost Alex we felt so alone and couldn't relate to any of the groups organised to help you cope with such a loss. But we now know there are people out there in almost identical positions which although reassuring it is very sad that so many preventable deaths have occurred and that lessons are not being learned.

To sum our story up, when we knew things had gone wrong in Alex's care and as parents it's our duty to stand up and prove our son wasn't another statistic or 'just one of those things', a quote you hear all the time from people who see the world with blinkers on and if it hasn't happened to them it never happened at all. I would like to think that as a parent, if we had received excellent care with Alex and he would be here today going to school and causing mayhem like most little boys, I would be open minded enough to read this story told by someone else and not turn a blind eye and say the truth has to come out so that the future can move on in a more positive and more importantly more trusting path.

Appendix 2

Letter from James Titcombe to Dr Bill Kirkup, July 22nd, 2015 (sent by email)

Morecambe Bay Investigation Report

I am writing following the publication of the Morecambe Bay Investigation report.

Firstly, on behalf of my family and I, I would like to say a sincere thanks to you and the investigation panel for carrying out such a thorough review. I feel strongly that your investigation has finally exposed the truth relating to what happened at Furness General Hospital maternity unit and the consequences that these failures have had on the many families affected. I also fully support the recommendations in the report and I am very much encouraged by the government response last week

As you know, I do feel that the response to date from some of the professional organisations and senior midwifery leaders has not always been as appropriate and at times, has been quite defensive. If lasting changes are going to be made it is clear that sustained effort and leadership is going to be needed.

As we have discussed in the past, there are some aspects of the report that I remain unconvinced about. Whilst I would emphasise that

I fully agree with the vast majority of the conclusions, I also wanted to ensure that those which I remain unconvinced about are put on record.

My first area of concern remains around the interactions between CQC, PHSO, DoH and ministers relating to the trust, especially around the 2009/2010 period. Whilst I agree that your report has accurately described many systemic issues and problems within each of these organisations and the way they worked together (or rather didn't), I remain of the view that there must have also been an element of deliberate 'playing down' of the emerging extent of the problems at Morecambe Bay ahead of the May 2010 general election.

I do not think that the central issue here was the registering of the trust without conditions, but rather the fact that discussions between CQC and PHSO resulted in a decision not to investigate Joshua's case, which preceded the act of registering Morecambe Bay without conditions.

As just one example to illustrate why I remain concerned; when Ann Abraham was interviewed she said that she didn't investigate Joshua's case because she was already convinced of the systemic nature of the problems at the trust and didn't want to delay the CQC taking appropriate action.

However, only months later when I referred my complaint about the NWSHA to the Ombudsman, that complaint was rejected for the apparent reason the Ombudsman had come to the conclusion that other serious incidents at the unit were NOT related and didn't demonstrate systemic issues that should have triggered earlier action from the NWSHA.

It doesn't make sense to me that my initial complaint to the Ombudsman was rejected because the systemic nature of the issues were apparently already known and accepted, yet my second complaint to the Ombudsman (just months later) was also rejected, this time because the Ombudsman was of the view that other incidents weren't related and didn't demonstrate systemic issues. The rejection letter to this complaint stated: 'I hope this provides some small comfort that earlier incidents didn't represent missed opportunities to change what happened to Joshua'.

I fear that somehow the Ombudsman has managed to escape detailed scrutiny regarding these decisions and to this day, no external process has been allowed to look in detail at the decisions themselves and the basis on which they were made.

I also remain unconvinced by the explanation in the report regarding the Tony Halsall email to his Chair '...if I'm right then the CQC will cover off the Ombudsman'. I think this statement does have a clear meaning and that this is something Tony Halsall wrote because he had reason to believe it to be the case. The explanation offered in the report makes no sense to me.

An Ombudsman investigation in 2009 is very likely to have revealed at least some of the issues your report uncovered in 2015. The truth about the failures at FGH (even in 2009) were deeply shocking and such public news would not have sat well within a DoH concerned about 'maintaining public confidence' ahead of an election and indeed, the depth and extent of problems might also have embarrassed a regulator that has since been criticised for having a preoccupation with its own reputation around this time.

There was thus, in my view an alignment of convenience whereby it suited everyone involved to act in a way that kept the bad news quiet. This I am sure, was at the heart of why the problems at Morecambe Bay did not attract robust external intervention sooner.

I accept fully that during the course of your investigation you didn't find conclusive evidence that supported this view. However, my view is that this is not in the least surprising as such circumstances are seldom exposed by people volunteering information. It is also regrettable that the details of how the Ombudsman reached the decisions made in relation to Joshua's case were not scrutinised. For example, the case advisor that worked on the case and recommended an investigation was not interviewed.

In my view, in order to rule out these concerns conclusively, a much more robust process of investigation was needed around these specific issues.

I should emphasise again that these issues relate only to a small section of your report. The extent to which they matter is debateable. For example, I think that concerns about the 'no bad news' culture within the DoH and wider system are well known and broadly accepted by most informed people involved in healthcare.

I will finish by repeating that I remain supportive of the vast majority of the Morecambe Bay Investigation report and grateful to you and the panel for all your hard work. I am convinced that the recommendations are the rights ones and will make a huge difference to patient safety across the NHS.

Acknowledgements

Over the last 6 years I've been lucky enough to meet some wonderful people. It is not going to be possible to thank everyone here, but I must mention some.

A special thanks is owed to Carl Hendrickson, Liza Brady and Simon Davey for their courage and support, without which the Morecambe Bay investigation would not have happened.

I would like to thank DCI Doug Marshall, Christina McKenzie, Kay Sheldon, Paula Sparks, John Woodcock and Tim Farron for helping to stand up for the truth.

I also need to say a special thanks to Peter Walsh, Katherine Murphy, Vicky Jagger, Phil Hammond, Shaun Lintern, Charlotte Leslie, Will Powell, Kim Holt, Suzette Woodward and Julie Bailey for the considerable help and support they have provided over the years.

This book owes its existence to my dear friend Helen Hughes, whom I have learned so much from and whose support and encouragement have been invaluable.

I must also thank my mother and father, who have been with me on every step of this journey and my wife for being so strong throughout.

I would also like to thank Jeremy Hunt for listening to Joshua's story and promoting patient safety.

Finally, a huge thanks to Murray Anderson-Wallace, Anne Wallace and Roland Denning for all their encouragement and careful editing of the manuscript.

Index

236

237